"Ten tips to improve the nutrition, health and happiness of infants, children and adolescents."

"…Come, my friends,
'tis not too late to seek a newer world.

Alfred Lord Tennyson, author of the poem "Ulysses" 1833

ACKNOWLEDGEMENTS:

I would like to thank my husband, Alan, and my son, Jason, for their thoughts and patience while I wrote this book. I would also like to thank my late parents, Harry and Jessie, my late older brothers, Alan and Ronald and my late sister-in-law, Leah, who made me start to wonder when they all passed away, one by one … "what went wrong?" I want to thank my professors in the MS Integrative Nutrition program (a program that integrates medicine, and classical nutrition which is based on herbs and plants, with modern nutrition), giving me new understanding and my professors in the MS Biotechnology program (a program that trains students to use knowledge of Biology as a tool to improve health and wellbeing). I also want to thank the many families that have welcomed me into their home to care for their children on a part-time basis, as a back-up caregiver, allowing me to get hundreds of views of families in real-time, especially their food pantries and kitchens, while I fed their children snacks and meals. And, last but not least, I want to thank you, dear reader, for taking the time to read this book.

DISCLAIMER:

Please note that this book is not a substitute for medical advice. It is not intended to diagnose or treat any condition or disease and that concerns of a medical nature should be brought to the attention of a qualified medical professional.

Table of Contents

INTRODUCTION:

I am writing this book after raising my own child and also caring for hundreds of other children as a back-up caregiver. This work puts me in different families, sometimes every day. I have encountered healthy children, gifted children, average children, and some, less than perfectly healthy. While there are some things that diet and lifestyle can't change, an improved diet and lifestyle may help any child do their best and get the most out of their life.   It has been so striking to me to see what the children are fed, sometimes very nutritious and sometimes not. It stimulated a curiosity in diet and lifestyle and prompted me to pursue and complete a graduate degree in nutrition. I know that time is of the essence in families and they may feed their children with well prepared meals or, at times, hastily prepared meals and snacks, some consisting of highly processed foods. I did this, too, at times. These 'convenience' processed foods are often high in sugar, salt and saturated fat while at the same time, low in fiber and nutrients. Most parents want the best for their child and will do everything they can to give them the best chance at a good, healthy life. Knowledge of nutrition is therefore of utmost importance so that children are not short-changed of the essential nutrients they need at this important time in their lives. While I understand that it is every parent's choice what they feed their child, with knowledge, I believe that parents will make the best choices.

I was amazed to learn that it is a good practice to "eat the rainbow", that is, to include fruits and vegetables of many colors, because these different colored fruits and vegetables contain different plant nutrients (called "phytonutrients"). In addition to the vast array of vitamins and minerals that are present in these foods, here are some examples of these pigment phytonutrients: anthocyanins are found in the blue and purple foods such as eggplant, purple potatoes and blueberries; lycopene is found in red foods such as tomatoes, watermelon and red pepper; beta-carotene is found in the orange foods such as pumpkin, cantaloupe, and carrots; lutein in green and yellow foods such as corn, kale, spinach, lettuce, green pepper and yellow onion; flavanol is found in white/pale yellow foods such as cauliflower, garlic, pear and white onion. These are not just pretty colors; these phytonutrients have been shown to reduce our risk of several diseases, such as obesity, cardiovascular disease (CVD) and cancer. Also, anti-inflammatory and anti-oxidant compounds such as turmeric and polyphenols (found in berries, avocados, cocoa, nuts and seeds) may help us to slow the aging process caused by oxidative damage to our cells, improving our cells' physiology. Another happy result of eating fruits and vegetables is happiness since there are studies showing the consumption of fruits and vegetables can improve emotional well-being and creativity along with a decrease in psychological distress .[1,2,3] In one smartphone-based study, fruit and vegetable consumption contributed one quarter of the total eating happiness. [4,7] While studies on nutrition and nutrients are often observational, which is not the best kind of study, still, there have been some that are more rigorous, such as randomized controlled trials (RCTs) (the gold standard) and case-control studies that have been collected and reported on as reviews. [5,6]

I have learned a great deal on how our food affects our health, and I would like to share what I have learned with those readers who are interested in the relationship of food and health, especially in children. Also, studies show that nutrition in our growing years affects our health in adulthood, too. So, our adult health is also affected by our childhood nutrition.

I also have my own family story that prompted me to look at nutrition in more depth. I was still in high school when my dad got sick. He was diagnosed with Crohn's ileitis, an inflammatory bowel disease. I was in college when he passed away, from metastatic cancer. He was not yet 58 years old and I was devastated. But, I still had my mom and two older brothers. We were all pretty healthy, or so I thought, a little overweight, maybe, that is all. But, when my mom was in her 60s or 70s, (I am not sure because she did not tell me) she became a diabetic. She was an active person, singing in a choir, dancing on the weekends. Diabetes was in her family, she knew, since her mom and sister had succumbed to the disease. Somehow, though, she went on with her life until her late 70s, when one day she had a massive stroke. Her good friend found her on the floor of her apartment, unable to get up. It took everything – she could not walk anymore and had to move to a nursing facility. She lived there for over two years and in that time both her legs were amputated above the knee, due to diabetes and the resulting complications. We buried this dancing lady, age 81, without her legs, and again I was devastated.

After mom passed away, my oldest brother started to talk about his diabetes. He had already had double by-pass surgery, a secret until now. Now, diabetes was robbing him of kidney function which required kidney dialysis, and he had to have several toes amputated, too. He passed away a few months after his 62nd birthday. My older brother lasted a few more years and then he, too, succumbed to metastatic cancer, not yet, 62. I am the last living member of my childhood family, a witness to this devastation. My sister-in-law lasted a few years after her husband, and then she also succumbed to cancer, not yet 65. How could they be so sickly? What, if anything, could have prevented this? Looking back at our daily lives and diets when I was a child in this family, there was the Standard American Diet (SAD) as in so many families. We had some vegetables, maybe some iceberg lettuce and tomato, and fruit such as melon and apples. There was red meat, potatoes, and lots of processed foods such as boxes of mashed potatoes, pasta, and highly processed, sugary cereals. There was not much fish, no tofu, beans or nuts, and vegetables were a "side dish" not the main dish. The Mediterranean diet was not known, really, outside of the Mediterranean, certainly not in my home. Also, we were not an athletic family: Dad liked to lay on the couch and read, my brothers were interested in music and electronics and I was exercising, maybe once a week at most, after school and homework.

I know, also, that none of us three children were breastfed. This was a time (1950s) when formula feeding was being encouraged and breastfeeding was "not convenient," as my mom told me. I don't fault my mom for the fact that the American culture at the time did not encourage breastfeeding, except for maybe the small group of women who started the La Leche League, in 1956. [1] They simply did not know how powerful this liquid nourishment is for an infant.

So, I wish to impart to you, dear reader, what I have learned on this important topic, infant, child and adolescent nutrition, and how it affects their health as children, adolescents and in to their future.

BACKGROUND:

This book on the topic of nutritional and lifestyle changes that could benefit children comes at a time when there is a worldwide epidemic of childhood obesity, where childhood diabetes (traditionally seen in older adults, "late-onset") is becoming rampant, and where nonalcoholic fatty liver disease (NAFLD) is becoming more frequent in children, especially in overweight and obese children and adolescents. [1] In well-designed scientific studies, a picture emerges of the interplay between nutrition and health. This book is written for parents and caregivers as well as adolescents, who want to understand this relationship and how they can use it to their healthful advantage. I want to find ways for children, as they grow older, to use knowledge that they have acquired to scrutinize labels and provide self-care. If there is less-than-healthy food in the vending machine at school or they have to make choices in the pantry at home, they need the knowledge to be able to make an informed choice.

METHODS:

The question of what is making these diseases increase dramatically and what nutritional and lifestyle changes can be done is the focus of this book. The searches for pertinent studies were performed in the public database of scientific literature known as PubMed,[2] a repository of biomedical and clinical research publications. The randomized controlled trial (RCT) is the gold standard in clinical research, and is the source of the information, when available. This type of clinical trial is ideally double blind (which means the participants and the researchers do not know who was randomly assigned to which group until the end of the study), but since double-blind is hard to do in nutrition studies, other methods are useful, such as a placebo-controlled study (which means there are proper controls for the study such as no changes to their diet (control) compared to changes in the diet (intervention)). The window of time for studies to be included was 20 years, to make this information up to date, as of today.

I also have found other studies informative and helpful for writing this book, such as a prospective cohort study, (a study that looks ahead in time at a group of people, monitoring them as they go along) an example of which looked at the measurements of a fetus as they grew when the mom took DHA (omega-3 fatty acid) supplements beginning in the first trimester, and also case-control studies, which are again, two groups, dietary intervention (case) and no intervention (control), but not double blind or randomized. Some information was also taken from reviews, which bring together several studies. There are also systematic reviews, which systematically review papers, removing duplicates, or those that do not satisfy a list of criteria, and then use the remaining papers to answer a question. I have used these sources, as well, when they have information of interest to this topic.

CHAPTER 1: THE NUTRITION FACTS PANEL

We are fortunate to live in a time and place where food labeling is mandatory in order to aid consumers in making wise choices at the grocery store. In the US, the Nutrition Labeling and Education Act was enacted in 1990 and the Food and Drug Administration (FDA)) was given authority over the labeling and the nutrients to be listed. [1] This action came from increased scientific knowledge about the relationship between health and diet, and consumers wanting more accurate information. The Daily Reference Values (DRVs) were first established for reporting by the 1988 Surgeon General's Report on Nutrition and Health and the National Research Council's (NRC) 1989 report, "Diet and Health: Implications for Reducing Chronic Disease Risk." [2] The Daily Reference Value (DRV) for fiber at that time, for example, was given as 10-13 g/1000 calories, while the other nutrients were given in % of calories, such that they should add up to 100%. These were based on a 2000 calories/day diet (e.g., an average adult). There was no recommendation given for sugar. The nutrition label itself was the product of contributions from public hearings and focus group sessions, which were supporting a format that would be simple and understandable. The result was numeric values rather than bar graphs and pie charts, with quantitative amounts given for the macronutrients (fat, carbohydrate and protein). These values
were meant to allow the consumer to determine quickly if the food contained a lot or a little of a nutrient. Eventually, the FDA worked with graphic designers and, with guidance from research findings, created designs for easy comprehension. The

labels are constantly evolving based on new nutrition information.

Do parents and caregivers know how to read these labels, what to look for on them and how to respond to the information? Can an adolescent read them and understand them? We can look together at this important Nutrition Facts Panel (NFP), and you can learn how to use them to your advantage. Looking at the new nutrition facts label, [3] the serving size and calories are now in the larger, bold font. The daily values have been updated, and added sugars, vitamin D and potassium are now included in the list. Added sugars were added to the label in 2016, to distinguish those sugars that are naturally present in the food. Some serving sizes and daily values (reported in % of daily value) have been updated. Here is an example of the current Nutrition Facts Panel from the website www.fda.gov (2022)[3]:

Nutrition Facts

8 servings per container
Serving size   **2/3 cup (55g)**

Amount per serving
Calories   230

	% Daily Value*
Total Fat 8g	**10%**
Saturated Fat 1g	**5%**
Trans Fat 0g	
Cholesterol 0mg	**0%**
Sodium 160mg	**7%**
Total Carbohydrate 37g	**13%**
Dietary Fiber 4g	**14%**
Total Sugars 12g	
Includes 10g Added Sugars	**20%**
Protein 3g	
Vitamin D 2mcg	10%
Calcium 260mg	20%
Iron 8mg	45%
Potassium 240mg	6%

* The % Daily Value (DV) tells you how much a nutrient in a serving of food contributes to a daily diet. 2,000 calories a day is used for general nutrition advice.

(For educational purposes only. These labels do not meet the labeling requirements described in 21 CFR 101.9.)

Things to note here include
* The serving size, (2/3 cup), which can be compared to the
amount a person actually eats. It is given in familiar units such
as cups or pieces and in the metric quantity (55 grams).
* The number of calories.
*The nutrient facts listed give you information on this
particular food.
**It is recommended by the FDA that at least 100% of the
Daily Value (DV) be consumed each day of dietary fiber,
vitamin D, calcium, potassium and iron.
**In this example, the carbohydrate/fiber ratio is 37/4 grams=
9.25. I always look for foods that have a ratio of 5.0 or less.
Alternatively, since most Americans are not consuming
enough fiber, it is best to look for foods with at least 3 grams
of fiber/serving.
**For the less desirable components, saturated fat, sodium and
added sugars, it is best to stay below 100% of the Daily Value
each day.
*This section also tells you if the nutrient in a serving of this
food is low (5% DV) or high (20% DV).
*At the very bottom of this label is a footnote which explains
that the daily values are based on a 2,000 calorie per day diet.
It is very important for consumers to be able to interpret the
nutrition labels so that they can benefit from them with their
daily dietary behavior.[3] Hopefully, the 2016 revisions for the
NFP have made it easier to understand. However, there are
still some calculations that consumers will need to perform. If
one is on a diet of 1,500 calories per day, the 100% daily
values will be decreased to 75% of the values shown
(1500/2000 X 100 = 75%). For example, to get the % daily
value for fat on a 1500 cal. diet, first, write down the fat noted
and use that to calculate the 100% daily value: (8grams)/10% =

16

(80 grams)/100%. This tells me that 100% fat allowance for a 2000 calorie diet is 80 grams. Now, multiply this by 0.75 since 1500 calories is 75% of 2000 calories, which gives 60 grams. (80 X 0.75). This is the 100% daily fat allowance for a 1500 calorie per day diet. So, then, 8 grams/ 60 grams X 100 = 13.3%, and this number is the % daily value of fat in one serving of this food (2/3 cup or 55 grams of this food) on a 1500 calorie diet. If I eat two portions, then I have to double it to get 13.3% X 2 = 26.6% of my daily value of fat allowance on a 1500 calorie per day diet.

CHAPTER 2: ESSENTIAL FATTY ACIDS

Have you ever wondered how early humans acquired the building blocks to grow bigger brains? Omega fatty acids, such as docosahexaenoic acid (DHA) are considered a candidate for driving the modern human brain to evolve. [1,2] One study, based on excavations in South Africa's southern coast, suggests that early humans changed their diets during a glacial period from foraging of land plants and animals to relying on rich shellfish beds, when already somewhat highly evolved humans learned to take advantage of the spring tides, occurring bimonthly. This event is thought to have occurred between 123,000 and 195,000 years ago. The African coastal food chain was more reliable and richer than inland sources of fish and this richer source of fish, and this marine food chain could improve health, especially brain health, due to the high levels of omega-3 fatty acids in fish and in seaweeds.   Some scientists think this event occurred much earlier, in fact, as the animal brain likely evolved in the ocean and rocky shores beginning hundreds of millions of years ago and that it depended on compounds not found in abundance on land, such as iodine and DHA. Fish was part of the hominin diet for millions of years and many nutrients in fish (copper, iron, iodine, zinc and selenium) played a part in the evolution of the human brain. The evolution of the large human brain is thought to have depended on the land/water (coastal) border for an abundant source of DHA in the form of lake and marine life. [1, 2]

While fat is still debated in the scientific literature, trans-fats are unanimously considered to be unhealthy. [3] However, omega-fatty acids, also known as polyunsaturated fatty acids (PUFAs), are considered essential in our diet. This fact is because we do not make them due to the lack of the proper enzymes; thus, it is essential that we ingest them from our food.[4,5,18] The two main classes of essential fatty acids (EFAs) are omega-6 and omega-3. These fatty acids are distinguished by the location of the first carbon double bond (C=C) in the fatty acid chain. The omega-6 fatty acid, linoleic acid (LA) metabolizes to arachidonic acid (AA) while the omega-3 fatty acid, alpha-linolenic acid (ALA) metabolizes to the two active forms, eicosapentaenoic acid (EPA) and docosahexaenoic acid (DHA) in the liver. [29] Some omega-3 and omega-6 fatty acids are decreased in certain psychiatric diseases such as ADHD, bipolar disorder, depression, and autistic spectrum disorder (ASD). In particular, in children with ASD, lower levels of the omega-3 PUFAs EPA, DHA and the omega-6 PUFA, AA are sometimes seen, along with a lower ratio of total omega-3: total omega-6 PUFAs. The increase in the ratio of omega-3: omega-6 PUFAs in the Western diet could possibly reduce the incidence of these diseases. Studies at the molecular level, as well as anthropological and epidemiological evidence show that humans evolved in a much more balanced level of these essential fatty acids. This ratio has decreased over the past decades and has coincided with chronic inflammatory diseases. One theory is that the omega-6 PUFAs can convert to the pro-inflammatory molecule, arachidonic acid (AA) and can contribute to chronic inflammatory conditions while the omega-3 PUFAs are anti-inflammatory. [6, 28] The healthy ratio of 1:1 omega-6: omega-3 during human evolution has increased to 20:1 due to modern agriculture and food processing. The changes in animal feed, with emphasis on mass production has decreased the omega-3 fatty acid content in eggs (though sometimes ground flaxseed or flaxseed oil is added to feed to increase the omega-3 content in eggs, fish and animal meats). [7] This unbalanced ratio contributes to obesity and diabetes. A lower ratio is therapeutic with some diseases, too. [4,5,8]

Knowledge of dietary sources of omega-6 fatty acids and omega-3 fatty acids may help people at the grocery store. The omega-6 fatty acid is mostly found in grain-fed animals, eggs and dairy. There are variations, though. The egg yolk from free-ranging chickens eating their natural food of insects, seeds, vegetation and grubs, has a much lower omega-6: omega-3 ratio than a typical farmed egg, for example. [5] There are also omega-3 enriched eggs on the market today. [7] In other words, depending on what a chicken is fed, the omega-6: omega-3 ratio may be high or low. The omega-3 PUFAs are found in aquatic organisms, such as oily fish (mackerel, salmon, herring), and lean white fish (cod, halibut). [9] These marine sources provide the omega-3 fatty acids EPA, and DHA. The main source of the omega-3 fatty acid alpha-linolenic acid (ALA) is plants, such as seeds, (flaxseed, chia seeds) and nuts (walnuts) and in green, leafy vegetables. Also, microalgae and some microorganisms, such as fungi, contain the omega-3 PUFAs. In fact, marine algae are the main producers of long chain (LC) omega-3 PUFAs (e.g., DHA). This eventually transfers into the fats of marine animals and fish. A consideration, for those that choose fish over supplements or plant-based sources of omega-3 fatty acids, is whether to consume wild caught or farmed fish. [10,11] Farmed fish feed on whatever the farm chooses to feed them, while wild caught fish eat what they can find in the water. The farmed fish may contain less omega-3 fatty acids than the wild fish. [5] Dietary sources of omega-3 from fish are salmon, herring, halibut, sardines, trout, oysters, fresh tuna and mackerel. Of course, one also has to consider that seafood may contain harmful toxins such as organic mercury and polychlorinated biphenyls (PCBs) from pollution and so, up to

2 (6-oz.) servings of fish per week are recommended in the Dietary Guidelines for Americans (DGA)[27]. The fishes with the lowest mercury content are salmon, shrimp, scallops, catfish, and pollock. [12]

Healthy dietary sources of omega-6 include nuts and seeds (walnuts, pine nuts, almonds, sunflower seeds, pecans). Nuts contain more than just the omega-6 PUFAs, they are a nutrient-dense food, associated with many health benefits, including a decreased risk in all-cause mortality, decreased inflammation, and improved blood sugar regulation. So, unless your child has an allergy to tree nuts, they are a good choice for a healthful food. When paired with dried fruit such as raisins, they are a convenient and healthful snack, providing dietary fiber, health-protective bioactive compounds, vitamins (such as A, B, C, and E) and minerals (copper, iron, and zinc, for example). Dried fruits are similar to fresh fruits in that they have a low glycemic load (GL) and moderate glycemic index (GI) (see chapter 4). Nuts are a healthful source of both monounsaturated fatty acids (MUFAs) and polyunsaturated fatty acids (PUFAs) while also being low in saturated fatty acids (SFAs). Nuts are also a good source of omega-3 fatty acids (especially walnuts), vitamins, minerals, as well as omega-6 fatty acids. [22] So, a handful of nuts is a good choice for most children. The overconsumption of omega-6 from seed oils (mainly soybean, safflower, and sunflower oils from processed foods) along with a deficit of omega-3 fatty acids in the diet has possibly contributed to an increase in allergy and autoimmune diseases. [13] Algae such as chlorella, spirulina, and nori, red algae that is used to make sushi, as well as wakame (a brown algae), dulse, and kombu is also a good food source of omega-3 PUFAs. These seaweeds, or 'sea vegetables' are often used in Asian and Latin American cuisine. [14] I add them in soups and stews.

Some oils contain high amounts of the omega-3 fatty acid alpha-linolenic acid (ALA) such as canola, flaxseed, soybean and walnut oils). [6] ALA is a precursor for EPA and DHA, but the conversion is inefficient. Thus, long chain (LC) omega-3 fatty acids (EPA and DHA) are essential, which again means we must include it in our dietary intake. The omega-6 PUFA linoleic acid (LA) conversion to arachidonic acid (AA) competes with the omega-3 PUFA ALA for the enzymes that will convert it to EPA and DHA.[28, 29] It is uncertain at this time whether or not this will have an effect on the final amount of omega-3 fatty acids and the pro-inflammatory omega-6 AA in cell membranes. It is known that the levels of consumption of omega-6 fatty acids are higher than omega-3 fatty acids. [29] Nutritional approaches using dietary omega-3 fatty acids may be a good choice to improve insulin sensitivity, control of body fat and to control inflammation and blood pressure. It can also improve child health. [5, 18,29]

The sources of linoleic acid (LA), an omega-6 PUFA) include the sunflower, safflower, corn and soybean oils. LA converts to AA, the starting molecule for many proinflammatory molecules. It is also consumed in some fish, meat and eggs, preformed. But, are these omega-6 PUFAs always bad for us or do they have some benefit? As it turns out, there is some benefit. [15, 28] It appears that that they also are the starting molecules for some anti-inflammatory products. In fact, when randomized controlled trials (RCTs) were used to evaluate the PUFAs, they found that replacing saturated fatty acids (SFAs) with PUFAs, most of which were omega-6 PUFAs, lowered the risk of coronary heart disease (CHD). The results also show that substituting refined carbohydrates, such as white bread, white rice, white potatoes, and sugar with omega-6 PUFAs will reduce CHD. They are also associated, at adequate intakes, with better child development.[29] There is some genetic variation regarding a person's ability to convert

the plant-based PUFAs which suggests human adaptation to
varying dietary sources of PUFAs. [28] The recommended intake
is 5-10% of caloric intake, while higher intakes, up to 25%,
may also be beneficial. [15] Maybe one day we will see these
important omega-3 and omega-6 fatty acids content listed on
the nutrition facts label.

What about olive oil and coconut oil? These include
the omega-3 and omega-6 PUFAs, in various concentrations.
A recent study [16] compared butter, coconut oil and olive oil, in
a randomized controlled trial (RCT), where healthy adults
were randomly divided into three groups and asked to consume
50 g per day of one of these fats, for a total of 4 weeks. The
main outcome for this study was a change in the (bad) low-
density lipoprotein (LDL-C) in serum, along with various
secondary outcomes (total cholesterol (TC) and high-density
lipoprotein cholesterol (HDL-C), body mass index (BMI),
blood pressure (BP), fasting blood sugar (FBS) and C-reactive
protein (CRP)). The results showed a significant increase in
LDL-C with butter consumption compared with either coconut
oil or olive oil. Butter also increased significantly the
TC/HDL-C ratio and the non-HDL-C serum components while
the two oils, coconut oil and olive oil, did not. So, it would
appear that these oils, coconut oil and olive oil, would be good
choices. [17] However, coconut oil is 100% fat, 80-90% being
saturated fat while olive oil is mostly monounsaturated fat
(MUFA) and polyunsaturated fat (PUFA). When it is
processed from the coconut to coconut oil, some other studies
show that it is similar to butter, raising cholesterol levels in a
way similar to other saturated fats. [23.] So, I think olive oil is a
better choice. It has vitamin E, a powerful anti-oxidant, along
with some essential fatty acids, omega-6 and omega-3, as well
as (mostly) omega-9. Extra virgin olive oil (EVOO), in
particular, has many healthful components worthy of

consideration in a healthy diet. The benefits of consuming EVOO may include improved gut and immune health. [24]

What is the earliest need for the omega-3 long chain polyunsaturated fatty acids (LCPUFAs) for a child? When the child is still in the womb, supplementation with omega-3 fatty acid reduces early preterm birth and increases birth weight, birth length and head circumference. Pregnant women who took 600 mg/day-1000 mg/day DHA in the form of capsules beginning <20 weeks had fewer preterm births (<34 weeks of gestation) and shorter hospital stays compared to the women in the placebo group. [18,19] Still, earlier omega-3 supplementation (the 1st trimester) showed improved fetal abdominal circumference, fetal head circumference and fetal head diameter. [20]
Interestingly, DHA can also have a positive influence on the mother's health. A recent analysis found that pregnant women who received a dose of 800 mg/day of DHA had a lower heart rate, and enhanced cardiac autonomic (involuntary) control, when compared to women receiving the lower dose (200 mg/day). [21]

So, the essential fatty acids (EFAs), especially the dietary omega-3 fatty acid, DHA, are very important for the brain, the retina, and the visual cortex. Essential fatty acids are also involved in the function and synthesis of brain neurotransmitters. Importantly, most of the growth of the brain is completed by age 6 and the human brain is over 50% fat. As mentioned above, the omega-3 fatty acids are important during the fetal and neonatal period, as well. [25, 26]

CHAPTER 3: BREAST IS BEST

When I embarked on my studies in nutrition, I learned how important breastfeeding really is. As a mom who has breastfed my child, I know that breastfeeding is more work than adding the powdered formula to water and shaking it. I was attached to a breast pump at home and work, when I was not attached to my infant, and freezing what I could so that my husband could "breastfeed sometimes, too, letting me get some much-needed rest. I breastfed exclusively for the first six months and for a total of a year and a half, not as long as the current recommendation of two years. I wish I had done more.

Baby formula is more convenient than breastfeeding, but is it best for your baby? There appears to be abundant evidence that breast feeding is immune-protective and can confer lifelong protection against disease. While it is certainly more work and has challenges of its' own, such as sore nipples or the challenge of producing enough breast milk to support the infant, professional lactation consultants can help a new mother with these challenges so that she can provide breast milk, as much as possible. The result is an infant with improved chances for a healthy life, something every parent wants for their baby. Breastfeeding supplies much needed polyunsaturated fatty acids (PUFAs), for short) such as omega-3 and omega-6 fatty acids, which are crucial for good brain development of the infant brain and the visual system.

There are numerous articles that discuss at length the long- and short-term benefits of breastfeeding for both the mother and the infant. I will mention a few of them here. Most of the studies are observational studies because it is obviously unethical to randomly put infants in a "no breastfeeding" group for the purpose of research. An article on health outcomes for both the mother and infant notes that it is quite common for American women to start breastfeeding their infants (75%) but they are still not breastfeeding long enough to improve the health of both the mother and infant. [1] By the age of 6 months, about half of American infants are still being breastfed at all (44.3% in 2011) and exclusive breastfeeding in 2011 was 14.8%. In a more recent review, [2] the World Health Organization (WHO) concludes there are numerous benefits to breastfeeding including improved cognitive development, and a lower rate of obesity for both mothers and infants. There also are several chronic diseases that breastfeeding can help reduce in the mother including diabetes, hypertension, ovarian cancer, and cardiovascular disease. [3]

Worldwide, most infant deaths occur in poorer countries and breastfeeding can improve infant survival, protecting against the incidence and severity of pneumonia and diarrhea, which are the leading causes of death in children less than 5 years of age in these poorer countries. [4] There are the unique anti-inflammatory and immunologic components of human breast milk that protect the infant from infections. Together, these compounds transfer immunity from the mother to the infant, protecting the infant from many infectious agents, such as those that cause diarrhea and respiratory illness. The World Health Organization (WHO) recommends that breastfeeding be initiated within 1 hour of birth, that an infant is exclusively breastfed for up to 6 months of age and that breastfeeding be continued up to 2 years of age. In a review of breastfeeding worldwide, [4] it is estimated almost a million lives could be saved per year if near-universal breastfeeding were achieved. Furthermore, the benefits of breastfeeding last into adulthood and, as mentioned previously, also benefit the lactating mother. [4] Looking at global breastfeeding data, in 2020, 69% of infants were breastfed up to 1 year of age and

44% were breastfed up to 2 years of age. However, as noted above for American women, this percentage varies greatly by country and by region.

When I returned to work after my child was born, I was lucky to be working in a workplace that had a "mother's room" – a separate, private room in a women's restroom. It had a breast pump, a refrigerator to store breast milk until it was time to go home, and a sign-up sheet so that other mothers at work could share in this resource. If you are not in a similar situation, you might consider bringing your own battery-powered breast pump to work, with an insulated bag to store the breastmilk in after you have finished. In July 2019, the US Congress passed the "Fairness for Breastfeeding Mothers Act of 2019." This law requires public buildings to provide a hygienic, shielded space other than a bathroom that contains a working surface, a chair and an electrical outlet for use by members of the public who wish to express human breastmilk. What's more, all fifty states, the District of Columbia, Puerto Rico, and the Virgin Islands now have laws that allow women to breastfeed in any private or public location. [5] The legal barriers to breastfeeding are breaking down and it is now much easier to discreetly breastfeed in public places. On the internet, I have found wearable battery-powered breast pumps. [6,7,8] These pumps are described as "hands-free, hospital-grade performance," it fits neatly inside the bra, are quiet and discreet. I have not used these products, but I mention them here so that a new mother might consider them as a possibility. Breastfeeding is more work than simply buying a container of powdered formula, but it is worth the effort, and thanks to innovations such as these in-bra breast pumps, and new laws that have relaxed restrictions on breastfeeding it is even easier than when I was a new mom. If you are a mother that wants to make breastfeeding a reality for your infant, there are resources available to support you. You may need to learn the

mechanics from a lactation specialist. This specialist can help
you learn the proper positioning of the infant, and how to make
sure they latch on to the breast properly. Also, importantly, no
discussion of breastfeeding would be complete without
mention of an important organization, the La Leche League
International.[9] This organization began in 1956 with a group of
seven mothers who wanted to support breastfeeding women
and provide breastfeeding help. At that time, breastfeeding
was not widely practiced nor encouraged by the medical
establishment. Their book, now in its' 8th edition, "The
Womanly Art of Breastfeeding" can provide the information a
new mom may need. An infant or child can benefit from this
amazing nourishment through the combination of
breastfeeding at the breast and expressed breast milk.
One other important point to make is that the mother's diet
may affect some nutrients more than others. [10] Essential fatty
acids, now implicated in neurological development,
specifically the essential omega-3 fatty acid, DHA, are
exquisitely sensitive to the maternal diet. The omega-3 and
omega-6 fatty acids transfer from the mother's diet into the
human milk. Importantly, these essential fatty acids and other
nutrients implicated in neurological (brain) development, such
as vitamins B-6, B-12 and D, folate, and the minerals iodine
and selenium do vary according to the maternal diet.[10] In a
recent study, [11] those mothers that adhered to the
Mediterranean diet, a plant-based diet that includes a moderate
intake of fish and poultry, vegetables, fruits, cereals (high in
fiber and minimally processed), with moderate intake of dairy
such as cheese and yogurt, a moderate intake of nuts and
legumes, extra virgin olive oil (EVOO) as the main source of
fat (e.g. a high monounsaturated fatty acid (MUFA) to
saturated fatty acid (SFA) ratio) showed a lower content of
saturated fatty acids and a higher content of MUFA in the
human milk, and a higher content of the major types of omega-

3 fatty acids alpha-linolenic acid (ALA) eicosapentaenoic acid (EPA)) , docosahexaenoic acid (DHA), and docosapentaenoic acid (DPA). Also, it is important to keep in mind that human breast milk is best for proper development of the intestinal immune barrier.[12] The current dietary recommendations from the USDA for pregnant and nursing mothers is a modified MyPlate, [13] since an extra 500 calories per day during breastfeeding is needed, with this number increasing as the infant gets older. Added salt, caffeine, alcohol and sugar-sweetened beverages (SSB) are best consumed in limited quantities while foods that are high in antioxidants, iron and omega-3 fats are advised. Foods that are specifically recommended include greens, starchy vegetables, fruits, fortified cereal grains, calcium-rich foods and a variety of plant- or animal-based proteins while minimizing those seafoods that tend to be high in toxic levels of mercury. For those lactating women who wish to omit some or all animal products, fortifying with supplements is recommended. [14]

The formula option is a viable alternative if breastfeeding is not an option, which it may not be for several reasons. Importantly, powdered formula must be made with clean water, and in many parts of the world, there is inadequate sanitation. Also, while every effort to mimic breastmilk is made when producing an infant formula, including using cow milk or soy milk as the base, and adding supplemental ingredients such as iron, fat blends, and the essential fatty acids arachidonic acid (AA) and docosahexaenoic acid (DHA), along with (sometimes) probiotics, it is still not identical. [15] Soy plant-based formula has been used for over 100 years and improvements to the product quality have been made during this long history, making this an adequate and safe alternative to cow's milk formula for most infants. [16] Breastfeeding is important enough that the University of Rochester (Rochester,

NY, my undergraduate alma mater), established the Division of Breastfeeding and Lactation in the Summer of 2022, to promote and advance this very important cause. [17] So, the take-home message from all of this is to eat a healthy diet while pregnant and lactating (if at all possible) to give your baby the best chance at good health.

CHAPTER 4: GUT HEALTH, FIBER AND FERMENTED FOODS

This is a really important topic, especially in this day and age, with the processed snack foods that children are consuming regularly. Our health is determined in large part by the health of our gut microbiota, a collection of bacteria that have evolved to live in our intestines. Our gut health is affected by many things such as our intake of antibiotics,[1] whether we were breastfed or not, [2] and whether we spend time in nature where microbes live. [3] It is affected by our attendance (or not) in a day care setting [4] as those children in day care have a more diverse pattern of microbiota, similar to an adult. These bacteria can provide extra energy to us in the form of short chain fatty acids (SCFAs) that they produce from the dietary fiber and starches we are unable to digest ourselves. So, this relationship is symbiotic; it provides a benefit to both the bacteria and the host, it is important for our health and depends on a fair amount of fiber in our diets. The health of our gut bacteria can also affect our moods and immunity. Thus, dietary fiber is very important as it is protective against cardiovascular disease (CVD) and coronary heart disease (CHD). It is also important for reducing metabolic syndrome, (a disease defined as having a combination of abnormalities such as high blood pressure, high blood sugar, high cholesterol, high triglycerides and obesity), inflammation, obesity, and constipation.

Dietary fiber intake in children is one of the reasons I was prompted to write this book. When children eat a lot of low fiber foods, bacteria that live in the gut are not well nourished. In my own experience as a caregiver of young children, I often see fruits and vegetables, which are high fiber foods, mixed with or replaced by low fiber foods, such as crackers, cookies, cakes, breads, and cupcakes.

A rule of thumb for dietary fiber intake is that the carbohydrate:fiber ratio of foods should be 5:1 or less or that there is at least 3 grams of fiber in a serving of the food. This information is something easily seen on the Nutrition Facts Panel (NFP). In fact, most processed foods have a carbohydrate: fiber ratio that is much higher. They also usually have less than 3 grams of fiber in a serving. It is easy to check the labels to help find the highest fiber foods. There are several children's books that can also aid in a young person's understanding of the bacteria that live and work inside of us and how they help to keep us healthy. Examples include "Garden in Your Belly", "Gut Garden", and "The Incredible Microbiome". [7,8,9] There are some excellent books for getting children to try new foods, such as the classic, "Green Eggs and Ham", and "I Will Never Not Ever Eat a Tomato". [10,11] "The Berenstain Bears and Too Much Junk Food" is a way to discuss junk food. [12]

These bacteria can also be adversely affected by broad-spectrum antibiotics. Antibiotic use can cause a loss of diversity in the microbiome and can perturb the microbiome for years. Early-life antibiotics may be associated with an increased risk of chronic diseases, such as diabetes, inflammatory bowel disease (IBD), food allergies and juvenile arthritis, most likely due to disruption of the microbiome. There is also some early association between childhood antibiotic use, overweight and obesity. There are times when antibiotics are the best choice, but they should be used only when necessary. Due to an increase in our knowledge of the gut microbiome, in 2016, the Center for Disease Control (CDC) created guidelines for the use of antibiotics in the outpatient setting in order to become more responsible in prescribing antibiotics. [5,6] Inappropriate use of antibiotics includes unnecessary use (such as for viral infections) and less than optimal selection of the specific antibiotic, the dose and the duration of use. As observed with mice, changes in the gut microorganisms due to the standard Western diet or antibiotics during critical periods of development have a long-lasting impact on the microbiota and the host. [13,14] In a recent study with mice who were exposed to the standard Western diet during their 'juvenile' period, it reduced bacterial composition and diversity in the adult mouse intestine. The juvenile diet in mice, then, has a long-lasting effect on the health of the adult mouse. Importantly, a similar result is observed in humans, when comparing different diets from around the globe and the resulting gut microbiome (bacterial diversity and composition). [15]

Fiber originates from plant-based foods. They are non-digestible to us and there are two main types of dietary fiber. Soluble fiber comes mainly from fruits and vegetables while insoluble fiber comes mostly from whole-grain products and cereals. Most high-fiber foods contain, in varying amounts, both soluble and insoluble fiber. Dietary fiber is associated with a healthy metabolism, such as insulin sensitivity. Our gut microflora, the bacteria, ferment this fiber for us in the gastrointestinal tract, and produce short chain fatty acids (SCFAs) that benefit us in many ways. The risks associated with a diet that lacks sufficient fiber include a less than optimal metabolism and chronic inflammation.
There are many things that have contributed to the modern, fiber-impoverished diet. In the case of processed foods, the fiber has been largely removed during processing. Whole, unprocessed foods are thus a better choice. In addition, there may not be enough whole grains, fruits and vegetables in the diet, especially for young children. Since there is ample

scientific evidence that dietary fiber provides many health benefits, increasing dietary fiber is of utmost importance. A somewhat recent article focuses on the question of fiber in children and the effects of fiber (or lack thereof) on the health of children. [16] Here, there is discussion of the importance of increasing fiber intake to lower the risks, significantly, of diabetes, obesity, and constipation. At that time, (2012) fiber intake was recommended by the Institute of Medicine (IOM) in the following amounts: 19 g/day (1-3 years old), 25 g/day (4-8 years old) and 38 g/day (14-18, year old boys), depending on the age and gender. In 2015, the UK Scientific Advisory Committee on Nutrition gave somewhat similar results. [17] The quality or the source of the fiber is also important because different types of fiber have different physiologic functions and effects. There are variations in the degree that the fibers can be fermented and used for bulk, different compositions, and there is a need to understand what vitamins, minerals and phytochemicals are needed so that the fiber can be properly fermented by the enzymes of the gut bacteria. The discussion here, though, is how to get children and adolescents to consume enough of the proper fiber that they need. The SCFAs acetate, butyrate, and propionate are the major fermentation end products made by our gut bacteria, and they provide additional energy to us and strengthen our gut's barrier. [18] These microbes also add to the health of the host through the biosynthesis of amino acids, vitamins, and by affecting antibody expression.

So, foods that a parent or adolescent may want to consider including are, of course, vegetables and fruits, and unprocessed grains such as whole grain oats, and barley. The sweeter the fruit is, the more sugar it contains, so an unripe banana is a better choice than a ripe or over-ripe banana. The foods to consider excluding are highly processed foods that are low in fiber (less than 3 grams per serving), and foods high in added sugars since added sugar is non-nutritious calories. These are pieces of information that are found on the Nutrition Facts Panel (NFP) on the package.

Let's take, for example, white rice. Some families eat rice several times a day, and in many cultures, that is white rice. A better choice is the whole grain, brown rice variety, in small amounts. After processing, the white rice has lost the fiber, vitamins, plant nutrients that include antioxidants, and minerals. It also has a higher glycemic load (GL) due to the loss of the fiber. So, what is the glycemic load? It is the glycemic index (GI) of a food times the amount of that food where the (GI) is a rating for each food containing carbohydrates. The GI rates how much that food will affect blood sugar levels and the higher it is, the greater this effect on blood sugar levels will be. In this case, the whole grain, brown rice has a slightly lower GI value than the white rice but it is still best in small amounts because it still has carbohydrates and thus a high GI and glycemic load (GL). Thus, the high-carbohydrate foods that will generate the biggest spike in blood sugar are highly refined, with most of the fiber removed, such as white pasta, white rice, white bread, sugar-sweetened beverages (SSBs) and highly processed foods and cereals. Low-GI foods (55 or less) include fruits, dairy products and legumes. [19] In addition, different ways of preparing a food may change the GI of the food. Sweet potato has a lower GI when boiled than when it is roasted or baked. [20] Several lists of GI and GL are available online to help guide a person to healthful eating.

Returning to the topic of fiber and the health of our gut bacteria, it appears that a large change in diet, such as going from an animal-based to plant-based diet, can rapidly change the gut microbiota.[18] There are basically two kinds of carbohydrates, digestible (to us) and non-digestible. The digestible carbohydrates include starches and sugars, such as glucose, fructose, lactose, and sucrose. They are degraded by enzymes in the small intestine of the gut and glucose is released into the bloodstream which will stimulate insulin. The non-digestible carbohydrates include resistant starch and fiber and are not degraded by enzymes in the small intestine of the gut. Instead, they travel further down to the large intestine (the colon) where they will be fermented by the microorganisms that live there. In this way, the microbes will provide the host with energy, in the form of short chain fatty acids (SCFAs) such as butyrate. The fibers are prebiotics ('food for the gut bacteria') which are defined as the non-digestible parts of food that benefit the host by selectively stimulating the activity and/or the growth of gut microorganisms. The sources of these fiber prebiotics include soybeans, raw oats, and unrefined wheat and barley. Diets that are rich in these non-digestible fibers results in a healthier gut microbiome. In contrast, diets that have reduced fiber intake and a consistently lower production of SCFA are less healthy and this low fiber diet has been noted in colon cancer patients. [18] An imbalance between good and bad bacteria, with a net reduction in short chain fatty acids (SCFAs) production, are associated with various gastrointestinal diseases such as inflammatory bowel disease (IBD), irritable bowel syndrome (IBS) and colorectal cancer. In addition, diet-induced gut imbalance of good (protective) and bad (pathogenic) bacteria appears to be a contributing factor in nonalcoholic fatty liver disease (NAFLD), obesity and diabetes, certain cancers, chronic inflammatory bowel diseases and other immune disorders, all diseases that young people can get. [21,22] These protective organisms that live in our intestines protect against invading pathogens' ability to colonize the gut by using SCFA to regulate virulence genes. If you think of the microbiome as a 'garden' or 'ecosystem', the goal is to weed out the bad microbes, and then to seed and feed the good microbes. And, a healthy individual will have a highly diverse microbiome while a less healthy or diseased individual will have lost this diversity. [23] This low microbial diversity is observed in people with obesity, type 2 diabetes, and also inflammatory bowel diseases. The more diversity in the diet, the more diverse will be the microbiome, making it able to respond to physiologic needs and challenges that affect metabolism such as the state of energy intake, and digestion. Pre-adolescent children are trying new foods and thus may have a more diverse microbiome than their parents. Habitual diets, established by adulthood, result in a personalized gastrointestinal (GI) microbiome. What can we do to improve our microbiome? Dietary changes can alter our microbiome in as little as 3 days. For example, trimethylamine (TMA), made by intestinal microbes when foods such as red meat, poultry, eggs, milk and shellfish are consumed, can be oxidized to trimethylamine-N-oxide (TMAO), associated with atherosclerosis (hardening of the arteries). However, the addition of foods common to Mediterranean diets, such as extra-virgin olive oil (EVOO), grapeseed oil, balsamic vinegar and red wine can inhibit TMA production. [23] These gut bacteria can help us to get the most out of our nutrients and energy by maximizing their absorption. In addition to the main determinants of gut microbiota composition, genetic and environmental factors, diet can affect the bacteria in the intestine and also microbial fermentation. For example, studies show that dietary polyphenols, which are widespread in the plant kingdom, may help maintain the balance of gut microbiota. Polyphenols are found in cocoa, tea, wine and common fruits and vegetables. [22] Most dietary polyphenols are not absorbed in the small intestine and are instead metabolized in the large intestine (the colon), where they are acted on by the bacteria of the colon. The beneficial effects of these dietary polyphenols are mostly due to the breakdown products derived from the activity of the gut bacteria. Thus, these polyphenol-rich foods, such as wine, green tea, coffee, cocoa, apple and grape extracts, have been found, at least in animal studies, to increase the degree of biodiversity of intestinal bacteria. Also, in the presence of these foods, good bacteria, such as *Bifidobacterium,* increased and bad bacteria, such as *Clostridium,* decreased in number. [22]

I wanted to get a better understanding of polyphenols and to provide it to you, the reader. These plant chemicals help to protect the plant from damage due to pathogens and UV radiation, for example. They also confer the vibrant colors on fruits and vegetables. And, they are one of the two main groups, along with short chain fatty acids (SCFAs), the product of fermentation of the non-digestible carbohydrates found in dietary fiber, that influence several functions of the human body. These influences are due to the release by the gut bacteria of bioactive molecules and their absorption into circulation. Fiber also is a source of polyphenols. The polyphenols we eat are degraded by the microbiota and these are made highly bio-available to us by this degradation process. This improved bioavailability allows the products of polyphenol degradation along with the fermentation of fiber to offer us a range of health benefits .[24] So, you may want to keep these high fiber foods in mind, especially at the grocery store. For more complete lists of these high fiber foods, go to the National Library of Medicine. [25]

A discussion on gut health would not be complete without the subject of fermented foods. There are many fermented foods to choose from, such as kombucha, yogurt, kefir, fermented cabbage ('kimchi'), sauerkraut, fermented carrots and fermented fish, such as herring. Why, you might ask, is that important here? Well, it turns out our gut microbiome is positively influenced by both plant-based high fiber foods (fruits vegetables, grains, nuts, seeds and legumes) and fermented foods. In fact, a recent comparison study found that only the high fermented food diet both decreased markers of inflammation and increased the diversity of the microbiota in the gut. [26] The high fiber diet, while increasing the function of the microbiome, such as increasing the growth of bacteria involved in fiber degradation, the production of SCFAs and the enzymes for degrading complex carbohydrates, did not increase the microbiome diversity in this study. When new US immigrants adopt our Standard American Diet (SAD), there is a loss of microbial diversity and microbial functions, along with a rise in inflammation markers, hallmarks of deteriorating health. So, both fiber and fermented foods are emerging as healthy choices. I personally enjoy pickles (fermented cucumbers), fermented carrots, yogurt, and pickled herring. Children, too, can learn to enjoy these fermented foods.

CHAPTER 5: MINIMAL ADDED SUGAR

This is another topic that prompted me to write this book. I have walked into the homes of several families that are top-heavy with sugary snacks. It can be fun to make cakes, cookies and cupcakes, but, all at once?? Or, busy families, with lots of afterschool activities, but short on time, will hand out the cookies and sugar sweetened chocolate milk before they head out to an afterschool activity. Our food culture has sugar everywhere. It is on top of glazed donuts, in the birthday cake, in the candy bars and in most processed foods. It has many names, such as high fructose corn syrup (HFCS), organic and raw sugar, and there are sugar substitutes such as erythritol, as well. What we know about added sugar is that it is not a nutrient, even though we use sugar ourselves, in the form of glucose, for energy. Table sugar, or sucrose, is a combination of glucose and fructose. Sugar is often found in plants, such as sugar cane and sugar beets, which are then refined and are the source of added sugar used in most processed foods.[1] Table sugar is associated with tooth decay, and can increase caloric intake without the other important nutrients associated with natural sugars found in fruits and vegetables. These added sugars replace nutrient-dense foods in the diet, and can potentially lead to undernourished, yet obese children and adults. In particular, sugar-sweetened beverages (SSBs), a major source of dietary sugar, are linked to dental cavities, obesity, diabetes, high blood pressure, heart disease and sugar can increase the growth of tumors. In fact, due to their role in the growth of cancer cells, refined sugars are considered to be a major cancer-causing agent .[1] Both the World Health Organization (WHO) and the U.S. Department of Agriculture (USDA) recommend limiting added sugar to no more than 10% of daily calories. Nowadays, children consume around 16% of their total calories from added sugar and much of this, 40%, comes from sugar-sweetened beverages (SSBs). [2] Children love sugar in most things. So, the best thing to do may be to find alternatives to refined sugar that are not harmful to their health. Unrefined sugar from natural sources such as fruit contains many compounds that can decrease inflammation, minerals, fibers, bioactive compounds, phyto (plant) chemicals such as flavonoids, and anti-oxidants. One alternative to refined sugar is fresh dates, which are rich in dietary fiber, vitamins, minerals, and polyphenols. Grapes also have many bioactive compounds, which provide several health benefits including anti-oxidant, anti-inflammatory and anti-microbial activities.[1] Sugars are naturally present in raw vegetables and fruits so they may be useful to sweeten foods. Monk fruit, from a plant grown in China, has anti-inflammatory, anti-cancer and anti-obesity properties, along with other health benefits. Stevia leaves contain essential amino acids, antioxidants, dietary fiber, phenols and protein. They exhibit anti-inflammatory properties, and are safe to consume. Stevia extract is considerably sweeter (300X) than other refined sugars and thus can be used in smaller amounts when preparing food with it. Other natural sweeteners to consider are honey, unrefined sugar beets and unrefined sugar cane. [1]

What about non-nutritive sweeteners (NNS)? Saccharin and sucralose, studied for two weeks in a randomized controlled trial (RCT) were found to impair glycemic (sugar) response in healthy adults.[3] Stevia extract, also considered a non-nutritive sweetener (NNS) , e.g., providing a sweet taste with no calories, had no significant difference in insulin or glucose responses in young adults when compared to a control group of young adults (aged 20-30 years old) over a period of 12 weeks, but a difference in body weight was observed compared to the control group as the stevia group maintained their weight while the control group gained weight .[4] The stevia leaves and whole stevia leaf extracts have, in addition to the compounds that make it sweet, been shown in numerous studies to have health benefits, such as anti-inflammatory, antibacterial (especially those that cause tooth decay), anti-oxidant, antitumor, anti-diabetic and antihypertensive properties. [5] There was a note of caution that not all commercial products of *Stevia* are of high quality. However, high quality *Stevia* products are a high-potency sweetener, with no caloric value. My impression is that, whenever possible, it is better to stick to whole (unrefined) foods, plant-based, for sources of sweetener (e.g., whole fruit), and if possible, to limit sweets to one cup (for very young children, age 2-3 years) or two (for older children) of whole fruit per day. The 2020-2025 Dietary Guidelines for Americans suggest that added sugars should be limited to 10% of calories per day beginning at age 2 and that foods with these added sugars should be avoided for children under the age of 2. [6] The current estimates of the number of children ages 2-18 years of age that are below the minimum recommended amounts of fruit varies but it is significant and it can be improved by using whole fruit to sweeten their food, whenever possible. With so many delicious fruits to choose from, it should not be too hard to find some fruits that they enjoy. [7,8] Berries, including blueberries, cranberries, raspberries and strawberries, are especially healthy, are low in calories, and have been found to reduce the risk of some chronic diseases in adults, in particular, type 2 diabetes, cardiovascular disease (CVD) and inflammation. Berries contain vitamins and minerals, such as vitamins C, E, folic acid (vitamin B9) and K, and manganese. [9] They contain micronutrients such as anthocyanins (a type of flavonoid), polyphenols and tannins, which have been shown to exert health benefits, particularly, with diabetics. They provide dietary fiber (in the form of whole berries) and are low in sugar content. The best way to serve these berries is in the form of fresh, whole berries. Some processing methods, such as freezing and juicing, as well as storage duration and temperature, and also heating can decrease the anthocyanin content. Freeze-dried berries seem to effectively preserve anthocyanins in strawberries. The time of harvest (early versus late in the season) shows that summer strawberries have a higher phenolic compound composition. Organic blackberries also have a higher phenolic compound composition.

An important sugar to be aware of is high fructose corn syrup (HFCS). There is a process in our livers where high carbohydrate foods become fat in the liver. Beverages and foods that contain high fructose corn syrup (HFCS), a simple carbohydrate, are associated with the development of nonalcoholic fatty liver disease (NAFLD). This disorder can be a stepping stone toward liver cirrhosis and also is predictive of cardiovascular disease. Carbohydrates are turned into fat in the liver, a process called de novo ('new') lipogenesis ('fat generation') and contribute to NAFLD, more so than dietary fat. HFCS also increases the severity of NAFLD. Obesity, too, is linked with inflammation, insulin resistance (a precursor to type 2 diabetes mellitus, T2DM) and NAFLD. [10] When HFCS is used to sweeten beverages and they are drunk in a single large dose, rather than in small doses over time or eaten, the enzymes in the intestine cannot metabolize the fructose fast enough, and the result is it spills over, or moves to the liver.[11] Reducing fructose intake, from sugar-sweetened beverages (SSBs) table sugar and foods with added sugars, may reduce fat accumulation in the liver. [12] The Nutrition Facts Panel and the ingredients list should provide the information needed to make an informed choice.

CHAPTER 6: A HEALTHY LIFESTYLE

The topic of lifestyle encompasses many things, but here I am mostly talking about a daily diet. Is your diet low-fat, low-carb, vegetarian, Mediterranean, or keto? Does your diet include a lot of fiber and/or fermented foods? Is there a lot of added sugar or salt? What about alcohol? Is alcohol, in any quantity, good for adolescents, who might be drawn to it, through peer pressure? What IS the best diet for children, especially? I know this is an important topic with many different things to consider. I touched briefly on a comparison of diets in a previous chapter on gut health, where a study compared a high-fiber diet to a high-fermented foods diet. There, they found the high-fermented food diet resulted in a decrease in 19 markers for inflammation not seen with the high fiber diet. It was interesting, especially since fermented foods are not often included in a child's diet, except maybe yogurt. Referring again to the 2020-2025 Dietary Guidelines for Americans (DGA), one can see many good recommendations for the age 2-8, year old group. There are nuts, seeds and soy products, 2, 4 oz. equivalent/week and whole grains 1-3, ounce equivalent/day. Dairy is recommended at 2-2.5 cup equivalent/day. While dairy products are the main source of saturated fat in the American diet, there are also some important nutrients found in milk, such as calcium, potassium, and vitamin D. [1] For these three nutrients, milk was the main food source for children between the ages of 2 and 18 years. Dairy products can also provide protein, riboflavin, vitamin B_{12}, phosphorus, and saturated fatty acids (SFAs). Flavored milk and sweetened dairy products, such as fruited yogurts, can increase caloric intake, though. Modeling studies using the National Health and Nutrition Examination Survey

(NHANES) data from 2010 showed that when three diet scenarios were compared, (plant-based foods, protein-rich plant foods and dairy foods, such as milk, cheese, and yogurt), the dairy reduced the percentage of children that were not meeting the nutritional requirements, for several nutrients such as calcium, magnesium, protein, vitamins A and D. In particular, inadequate calcium and potassium intake could be improved with addition of dairy foods. However, in the American Medical Association (AMA) response, "Culturally Responsive Dietary and Nutritional Guidelines D-440.978" it is noted that lactose intolerance, while less prevalent in whites, often begins in childhood, and is common among many Americans, especially African Americans, Native Americans and Asian Americans. [2] For this reason, the AMA recommends that the DGA guidelines should mention that dairy products are optional, with a goal of eliminating barriers in schools to receiving alternatives to cow's milk. The Physician's Committee for Responsible Medicine also responded, stating that there are an estimated 30-50 million American adults that are lactose intolerant. [3] Lactose intolerance causes diarrhea, gas and bloating, due to a less than optimal breakdown of the milk sugar, lactose. The calcium in milk can be obtained in leafy green vegetables, tofu, cereal, and beans. The vitamin D in fortified cow's milk can be obtained from fortified cereals and grains, as well as sunlight, the natural source of this vitamin. Magnesium can be obtained from green leafy vegetables and legumes. Fortified plant milks, such as soy milk, oat milk and almond milk are healthful alternatives to cow's milk. A study of the mineral content of various kinds of plant-based milk was done in 2022 at the Institute for Food Safety and Health, by FDA researcher Ben Redan, Ph.D., and his colleague, Lauren Jackson, Ph.D. and it was presented at the Fall 2022 meeting of American Chemical Society. [4] Four essential minerals (which means we must get them from our food) which are not noted on the Nutrition Facts label, but are found in dairy milk, magnesium, phosphorus, selenium and zinc, were analyzed in several plant-based beverages, made from a single ingredient such as cashew, coconut, hemp, oat, pea, rice or soy. A total of 85 samples were analyzed, from a variety of brands. The statistical results showed that the mineral content varied between different types of plant-based milk alternatives and also between different brands of the same type of alternative milk product. Importantly, the results showed that two types of plant-based milk alternatives, (PBMA) pea and soy-based drinks had levels of these four essential minerals that were higher than cow's milk. The three minerals phosphorous, selenium and zinc, were found to be 50% higher in pea-based drinks. Another analysis looked at other micronutrients (calcium potassium, vitamin A and vitamin D) in PBMAs and found the nutritional content was mostly due to the fortification (addition) of the micronutrients (minerals and vitamins) and that for those that claimed to have amounts similar to milk, most of them did have amounts that were equal to or greater than the amount claimed. [5] When the product did not claim to be fortified, the micronutrient was undetectable or nearly undetectable. So, after a child is no longer breastfeeding or formula feeding, one might consider these alternative milks, important sources of these particular vitamins and essential minerals, especially if they have been fortified .[4,5]

When it comes to milk and the question of whether it is good or bad for children, unfortunately, there is conflicting information. At least one author summarizes milk consumption in the Western diet as a promoter of chronic disease.[6] This article mentions a group of hormones, including insulin, growth hormone and insulin-like growth factor-1 (IGF-1) that are stimulated by consumption of cow's milk and cow's milk protein. The abnormal stimulation of these hormones, by consumption of a cow's milk, can contribute to the epidemic in adolescent acne, as well as abnormalities in other organs. A study of overweight adolescents found IGF-1 increased with skimmed milk and casein (cheese protein) when compared to a control group, which drank water or whey (whey is derived from milk and separates from curds when cheese is being made) with no observed positive effect on growth after 12 weeks of milk-based drinks. [7] Others, as mentioned previously, show that milk is an excellent source of important nutrients that are often in short supply in the diet. I think it is important to note that there are several other sources of these important nutrients that are in short supply. The nutrients are the important thing. Calcium is found in tofu, tempeh, beans, (especially white beans and chickpeas), seaweeds, dark leafy greens and plant milks while iron can be found in legumes, nut seeds and leafy greens. Also, importantly, when iron-rich plant-based foods are paired with vitamin C-rich foods, such as orange juice, there is an increase in iron absorption from these plant-based foods. If one is to follow a completely plant-based diet, however, which does provide many health benefits, it is important to include fortified foods, nuts, seeds and supplements for various micronutrients (vitamins, minerals) and algal omega-3 fatty acids since studies have shown a completely plant-based diet is deficient in several of these micronutrients. [8,9,10]

A 2023 study, sponsored by the National Dairy Council (but not involved in data analysis) looked at adult mortality and dairy consumption and found no association between low fat and fat free dairy food and cancer or other causes (diabetes, heart disease) when comparing the lowest intake to the highest intake. Also, heart disease incidence was reduced with dairy food consumption, by 26%. [11] So, then, is dairy a good choice? It is still a major part of the American diet. It is recommended by the 2020-2025 Dictary Guidelines for Americans (2020-

2025 DGA) and the 2020 Dietary Guidelines Advisory Committee (2020 DGAC). However, a study done in 2014 had shown associations between other adverse health outcomes and animal protein consumption. Higher protein intake was associated with a 4-fold increased risk of cancer and diabetes, and a 75% increase in all-cause mortality in older adults (19 - 65 years old). These results were improved if the protein that was consumed was derived from plants. Consistent with other animal and epidemiologic studies, the findings showed that a diet rich in plant-based proteins will likely benefit all age groups. [12]

A more recent study (2022) looked at the relationship of dairy consumption during childhood and adolescence, an important period of time characterized by rapid growth, with later cancer risk. This meta-analysis, grouping together many observational studies, concluded that milk intake during the early years of childhood and adolescence might not have an association with higher risk of breast, colorectal and or prostate cancer. However, these authors also concluded that more studies are needed for a definitive conclusion due to the small number of studies that were included in this meta-analysis. [13]

I think that no discussion of dairy would be complete without talking about the use of antibiotics in dairy animals. Antibiotic use in animals is very common. Dairy cows get mastitis, a painful infection of the mammary gland; they also get foot infections, respiratory diseases and uterine infections. In the US, 80% of all antibiotic use is in animals used for food production.[14] Milk and milk products are used around the world for their nutritional and economic importance. The residues from the antibiotics, which are defined by the Food and Drug Administration (FDA) as "pharmacologically active substances," remain in the foods that are obtained from these animals. Tolerance levels of these antibiotic residues have been established for consumer protection. There is a National

Milk Drug Residue Data Base kept by the FDA and it reported a very small percentage (<0.01%) of milk product tests were above FDA tolerance levels. Yogurt and cheese may have antibiotic residues, but it may be inactivated slightly by heating, such as pasteurization. The biggest concern here is the emergence of antibiotic resistance and its' ability to spread. The use of these antibiotics can apply a selective pressure on the bacterial population to become resistant and when these resistance genes are acquired they may pass these resistance genes on to neighboring members of the population. Antibiotic resistance that is acquired either from consumption by dairy cows or by our own consumption (such as during an ear infections) of antibiotics is already compromising the ability of these antibiotics to treat life-threatening diseases in humans. So, then, the presence of antibiotic residues in the food chain can possibly result in the acquisition of transferable resistance genes to pathogens and can possibly result in serious infectious diseases. However, the published data that shows a link between the antibiotic residues in milk and dairy products and the emergence of these antibiotic resistant bacteria is inconsistent. Further, other factors may contribute to antibiotic resistance in milk bacteria such as the environment and milk processing practices. In addition, there are other toxic effects such as an allergy that these antibiotic residues may cause. They may also affect the composition and function of the gut bacteria. It is known that antibiotics at therapeutic doses can alter the gut bacteria along with the immune and metabolic health of the host. There have not yet been good quality studies done to look at the impact of the antibiotic residues in specific foods such as dairy products and milk on the human gut bacteria. Now, thanks to new molecular techniques, it is possible to detect the same gene in different samples, such as humans, animals and food and, in this way, some of the antibiotic resistance genes that have been identified in food bacteria have been detected in the human gut, thus providing indirect evidence that this transfer can happen. While one study has shown similar antibiotic resistance genes in humans and poultry meat, a similar study has not yet been done for dairy. So, while there is still more work to be done on the question of antibiotic use in dairy animals and the effects it may have on the milk produced and the people who consume it, it is best to be aware of the issue. [14]

In the 2020-2025 DGA section on protein foods, DGA recommends 2- 5 ½ ounce-eq./day. This recommendation is also described in weekly amounts: 10-23, ounce eq./week of meat, poultry and/or eggs, 2-3 ounce-eq./week of seafood/week and (as mentioned before) 2 ounce-eq./week of nuts, seed, and soy products for children age 2-8 years old. However, there are known risks to certain protein products, such as processed meat, that we should all be aware of. Processed meats, such as deli meat and hot dogs, are associated with a moderately higher risk of CHD (coronary heart disease) when one serving is consumed per day while one serving of plant protein sources, such as nuts, soy and legumes (peas, lentils) were associated with a moderately lower risk of CHD. This study was in adults. [15] That same year, 2020, an article addressed the question of how strong the evidence is linking red and processed meats to health risks.[16] In this review, it is noted that applying a rating system for large amounts of data from nutritional studies, (NutriGRADE), there is a positive association between consumption of red and processed meats and type 2 diabetes, and that this evidence is of "high quality" along with a "moderate quality" association between red and processed meats and mortality. In a strong statement, the authors of this paper state that there is considerable evidence from long-term studies that has demonstrated that diets high in red and processed meats (where processed meats are defined as meats that are transformed by smoking, salting, curing or fermenting to improve preservation or to enhance flavor) are associated with increased risks of cardiovascular (heart) disease (CVD), type 2 diabetes (T2D), cancer, (especially colorectal cancer) and all-cause mortality.[16] However, in the literature, there is still controversy surrounding red meat. [17] While meats contain vitamins, minerals, and amino acids, other effects, such as cooking techniques and processing such as salting/smoking for preservation, can affect these nutrients. [15,16] The iron in red meat, called heme iron may cause oxidative stress and be related to chronic diseases such as colon and rectal cancers .[16] In excess, iron can form chemical oxidation products, such as hydroxyl radicals, that promote DNA damage (mutagenicity). Non-heme iron, found in plants such as leafy greens, fruits, nuts, seeds, and whole grains may be helpful. Specifically, these anti-oxidant-rich foods may be able to modify these heme-iron oxidative mechanisms. In other words, it is important to balance iron for health. Another possible explanation is that the gut bacteria compete with the host for the dietary iron and some of the pathogenic bacteria, such as *Salmonella* and *Shigella*, need iron for colonization and virulence. In contrast, some of the beneficial bacteria, such as *Lactobacilli,* do not require iron. So, one explanation for iron increasing the chance of colorectal cancer is by shifting the ratio of pathogenic to protective bacteria in the gut. A protective response by the body may be for the iron to be sequestered which can block access by the pathogenic bacteria to this iron. While these mechanisms and explanations may actually be occurring, I want to note here that there is not a total consensus in the scientific community. Some studies show stronger associations between red meat and/or heme iron intake and diseases such as heart disease, type 2 diabetes (T2D) and cancer than other studies. Also, there appears to be a stronger case for colorectal cancer than for prostate cancer, for example. [16,17]

Compounds produced by cooking meats, such as heterocyclic amines (HCAs), and N-nitroso compounds produced by heme iron in processed meat, are thought to contribute to this cancer-causing environment. The HCAs are formed at high cooking temperatures and/or long duration. So, reducing the temperatures and cooking for shorter times may be helpful. However, some studies undertaken to find a relationship between the high intake of HCAs and cancer incidence have not shown this relationship when compared to healthy people. Other studies have seen higher risks associated with large portions of well-done and charred meats cooked at high temperatures. Polycyclic aromatic hydrocarbons (PAH) arise when meat is prepared over an open fire and the fat and juices from the meat drip onto the fire, causing flames. These flames contain PAH, and they can stick to the meat surface. The PAHs can also occur when meat is smoked. Thus, in this way, high heat is related to potential oxidation and potential DNA damage (mutagenicity) by consumption of meat or meat products.   The high temperature cooking may also increase the levels of advanced glycation end products (AGEs) and these end products have been shown to increase inflammation and oxidation. [17,18, 19, 20]

The Mediterranean Diet (MD) has been shown in numerous studies to be beneficial for cardiovascular health. A low AGE diet is similar to the MD with fewer restrictions. The low AGE diet allows many forms of animal products as long as they are prepared with lower heat and high humidity than typically seen in the Western diet. The MD diet involves patterns of food intake. Specifically, the intake of certain foods and food groups, such as whole-grain bread and brown rice, fruit, vegetables, legumes, fish, and olive oil, are consumed based on the Mediterranean Diet Pyramid (MDP). Polyphenols found in colorful vegetables, and anti-oxidant vitamins are also emphasized since they are known to have anti-oxidant effects and improve blood vessel health.[18,19,20]

For children, resveratrol, a polyphenol found in grapes, is another anti-oxidant food choice. It has also been shown to have anti-inflammatory and anti-tumorigenic properties. In fact, in addition to grapes, resveratrol has been found in a variety of berries, in peanuts and several plants, as well as red wine. With typical dietary consumption, though, there is only a small amount of resveratrol intake. The studies that show promise with resveratrol are mostly laboratory studies with cells in culture and animals, and with the use of supplements. Resveratrol has a very good safety record, and it does help with acne and anti-aging when applied as a cream, so maybe the most promising way to use it is in a cream applied to the skin where high concentrations can be obtained to reduce skin lesions such as acne in adolescents and with skin diseases. [21,22]

The MDP was updated recently from the previous (2011) version and it now reflects environmental concerns as well as nutrition and health considerations. [23] When compared to the previous version, it emphasizes lower consumption of bovine dairy products and red meat, and a higher consumption of locally-grown plant foods and legumes. Still, importantly, it recommends that each country develop their own guidelines based on the MDP and their own food systems and based on their culture. Some of the highlights of this updated MDP are that vegetables should be consumed frequently, with a variety of colors to ensure a broad range of plant nutrients and that fruit should be the main form of dessert. Also, with less cooking, there is likely a higher retention of vitamins and with less fuel use, less environmental impact. Meals that are consumed daily should have (1) high fiber (at least 3 grams/serving) cereals, (2) vegetables and fruits, with (3) small amounts of legumes or beans. These three main groups are plant-based and have been found to be preventative for several chronic diseases, healthy weight management and reduced greenhouse gas (GHG) emissions and use of natural energy resources. Scientific evidence supports the idea that a plant-based diet can markedly reduce the use of land, water and resources and can reduce GHG emissions. In addition, the MDP highly recommends, as much as possible, fresh, seasonal vegetables and fruits, minimally processed, free, as much as possible, from chemical pesticides. Olive oil, especially extra virgin olive oil which is high in nutrients and resistant to high temperatures, is recommended for both dressings and cooking food. Both virgin and extra-virgin olive oil (EVOO) are a major part of the MD and components of EVOO have active compounds that have a positive effect on our genes and which can play a role in prevention of several diseases. [23,24] EVOO is made up of oleic acid, a monounsaturated fat (MUFA) as the major type of fat, along with a few others, both saturated (Stearic acid) and unsaturated (Linoleic and palmitic acids), vitamins and polyphenols. These ingredients found in EVOO contribute to the nutritional value of the MD, and reduce oxidation and inflammation that are precursors to diseases such as cardiovascular disease (CVD) and cancer. [24]

An interesting study looked at 10 specific dietary foods/nutrients to see how consumption (or lack thereof) these foods affect health and disease trends. [25] The results, derived from the National Health and Nutrition Examination Survey (NHANES), were based on published data, between the years 2002 and 2012 and were evaluated separately and/or in combination for demographics such as age, education, race and sex. Diet-disease relationships of 10 dietary factors included: high sodium, low seeds/nuts, low vegetables, low fats, low seafood-derived omega-3 fats and high intake of sugar-sweetened beverages (SSBs), unprocessed red meats, processed meats, low whole grains, and low polyunsaturated fats. The dietary factors were correlated with deaths from

heart disease, hypertension, stroke and type II diabetes. The
results for coronary heart disease, (CHD) for example, showed
that each of these dietary factors was suboptimal (either too
low or too high) and that high sodium, low seeds/nuts, high
processed meats, high SSBs and low seafood-derived omega-3
fats accounted for the largest numbers of estimated diet-related
deaths when compared to optimal consumption of these dietary
factors. For deaths due to type 2 diabetes, the largest numbers
of deaths were due to high processed meats, high SSBs and
low whole grains. For stroke, high sodium, low fruits and low
vegetables accounted for the largest number of deaths. In the
age group of 25-34 years old, suboptimal diet was associated
with a large percentage (64.2%) of the cardiometabolic deaths
discussed here. While this study excluded people under the
age of 25, you might wonder if this information has any
relevance to children and the food they eat. In fact, it does.
The food sources that are of concern because of their high
saturated fat (SF), sugar and/or sodium content and/or low
fiber content are (no surprise) sweet bakery products, sugar-
sweetened beverages, cured meats/poultry and pizza, for
children 2-18 years old .[1, 26] There is some evidence that
reducing foods that have limited nutritive value, while
encouraging those foods that provide nutrients that are in short
supply in the diet may reduce the risk of chronic diseases, such
as hypertension, obesity, and cardiovascular disease (CVD) in
the future. [25, ,26]

A recent study takes a look at 'children's food 'the
'kid's meal' or the 'kid's menu'. [26] These foods, unfortunately,
are often ultra-processed, high in saturated fats, sodium, sugar,
including SSBs and are limited in nutrients and fiber. A diet
that favors these foods can have long-term detrimental effects.
The idea that there is food for children that is distinct from
adult food originated during prohibition, when the sale of
alcohol was prohibited by the Volstead Act of 1919. During

this time, the restaurant industry tried to make up for lost liquor revenue by expanding their clientele to include children, creating menus that are palatable to them. A typical kids' menu will include such items as hamburgers, grilled cheese, hot dogs, french fries, macaroni and cheese, and chicken nuggets or tenders, along with sugar-sweetened beverages (SSBs), often along with toy incentives to go with these meals. There have been efforts to improve on the children's menu, such as *KidsLiveWell,* a voluntary program launched in 2011 by the National Restaurant Association. This program and more recent efforts have not seen significant changes, though, in the nutrient content of the meals, even those that are fewer than 600 calories, one of the criteria for at least two full-serving menu items of *KidsLiveWell.* Also, the sodium and saturated fat content are still excessive. But, one must ask, are children different from adults? Do they need their own menu? The conclusion today is that healthful food is the same for adults and children. [26]

While specific foods were not looked at, a study done in 2010 did look at childhood risk factors for cardiovascular disease on adult mortality. [27] Non-diabetic Native American children (average age 11.3 years) were assessed for body-mass index (BMI, a measure of obesity), blood pressure, cholesterol, and glucose tolerance to see if they could predict premature death. Children were followed for an average of 23.9 years. Those children with the highest BMI were more than twice as likely to die during this follow-up period. Those children with the highest glucose intolerance were almost twice as likely to die (73% higher) during this follow-up period. In addition, childhood hypertension (high blood pressure) showed a significant association with premature death. High cholesterol in childhood, however, did not appear to correlate with premature death.

Another review looked at Finnish children to ask and answer the question of what role childhood food patterns and/or specific nutrients have on cardiovascular disease (CVD) in adulthood. 3596 children between the ages of 3 and 18 were enrolled and food patterns were determined based on food habit questionnaires, along with 48-hour dietary recall interviews for half of them. The food patterns developed in childhood remain stable throughout life and there was an association with early risk markers for CVD. Those diets that had low intakes of vegetables and fruit were found to have elevated markers for CVD risk factors while diets with a high intake of vegetables showed increased arterial elasticity, a sign of decreased risk for CVD. The conclusion here, again, was that childhood nutrition plays a major role in CVD progression. [28]

Another interesting consideration is how children eat. Children need to learn to self-regulate, that is to listen to their internal cues that tell them when they are hungry and full. A review of this topic notes that there is a relationship between a caregiver's feeding style and a child's ability to self-regulate. [29] Also, there are specific actions that a caregiver can take that may help a child learn proper self-regulation. This article, from the journal of the American Heart Association (AHA) focuses on a behavioral approach for reducing obesity in young children. Specific traits have been identified that contribute to childhood obesity and weight status. These include eating when not hungry, emotional overeating, drinking sweetened beverages, eating in response to food-related stimuli and the inability to avoid eating after being satiated, while other traits have the opposite effect, such as eating more slowly, with fewer bites per minute, emotional undereating, food pickiness and attempts to restrain eating. Caregivers can affect a child's self-regulation, to some extent. Many children have an innate ability to maintain healthy growth by varying their food intake in the process known as *self-regulation*. This ability, however, can vary from child to child and it appears that some children are born with a better ability to self-regulate their eating than others. This fact may be due to other factors, such as maternal pre-pregnancy obesity, the maternal diet during their pregnancy and excess pregnancy weight gain, all of which are associated with a higher risk of obesity among the offspring. Caregivers can support this innate eating self-regulation, or they can negate it and trigger a deviation from it. A caregiver can help maintain good eating self-regulation if they allow a child autonomy, so that they can start and stop eating in response to their own hunger or satiation. At the same time, the caregiver needs to provide some structure, in the form of high food quality and variety, with less availability of calorically dense, nutrient-poor foods. There are, in fact, four feeding environments that have been identified: authoritative, indulgent, uninvolved and authoritarian. The best of these four is found be the authoritative, which supports child autonomy while also setting boundaries around the food. The strategies that authoritative caregivers use include reasoning, complimenting, and controlling the food environment (what foods are in the home, for example) making nutrient-dense food options readily available and then allowing the child to make their own selections. In addition, they set up mealtime routines, and allow the children to decide what and how much to eat. In this way, there is a high level of response to the child's cues, and this style is associated with an improved child dietary quality. So, in this way, setting up meal times and making high quality foods available, a caregiver best supports a child's eating self-regulation. Apparently, when a child responds to a parents' (authoritarian) attempt to control specifically what or how much they eat, they also stop self-regulating in response to their own appetite cues, responding instead to the parents' directives. [29]

CHAPTER 7: NUTRITIOUS FOODS

There has always been a question in my mind of how nutritious our foods are. Do they have the same nutrient content that they used to have when I was a child? Are they better, worse, or the same? Do I REALLY need supplements to maintain proper nutrient levels for my health?

As it turns out, I am not the only one who has wondered. In 2004, a study compared the nutrient levels of 43 crops, measured in 1999, to USDA nutrient studies from 1950. [1] The study showed big declines in the median concentrations of calcium, iron, phosphorus, protein and vitamin C. A study in 2009 concluded that there were up to 40% declines in the mineral content of fruits and vegetables over the previous five to seven decades. [2] And, an increase in carbon dioxide (CO_2) in the atmosphere in the last 30 years has reduced the concentrations of important minerals, such as calcium, iron, potassium and zinc in plants while, at the same time, increasing the ratio of carbohydrates to minerals in plants. [3] These minerals are important because they support the human immune system and improve intellectual ability. In the case of wheat, fortification with minerals such as iron and zinc are not effective due largely to the fact that these minerals are removed during the industrial processing of the whole grain.[4] One solution, though controversial, is genetic engineering of the plants. For example, a two gene engineering strategy in wheat, a crop that has had only limited success in improving the mineral content with conventional breeding, was able to increase zinc in the flour two-fold. Iron was redistributed by this process in such a way that the milled flour had a three-fold increase in iron. This is important because bread wheat is a staple globally and provides up to 25% of calories, so a low intake from the diet of these essential minerals contributes to malnutrition. [4]

In many places in the world, the question of whether to buy organic or conventional food may not be the right question. There are places here in the USA where the stores don't carry many fruits or vegetables, only processed, high-energy, low-nutrient foods. These are often referred to as "food-swamps" or "food-deserts", and they are found in poorer neighborhoods. There might be some canned fruits and vegetables to choose from, and that may be the best one can do. If you are lucky to have a choice at your local grocery store, you might wonder if it is worth the extra money to buy organic vegetables. I certainly have.

A 2021 study [8] notes that previous studies have shown there to be little difference in the macronutrient content (protein, carbohydrates and fats) of the crops but, at the same time, the micronutrient (nutrients present in small amounts, such as minerals) concentrations can be greatly affected by the farming practices and the plant variety. Also, conventional crops contain higher pesticide levels while the organically grown plants have higher levels of beneficial compounds that exhibit the protective anti-inflammatory and anti-oxidant capacity. These beneficial compounds, phytochemicals, are positively affected by farming practices that improve soil biodiversity. So, my impression is that, if you can afford it, there are some nutritional benefits to be gained by consuming whole, unprocessed, organic foods.

In an effort to get the best nutrition from foods, especially for children, what other foods besides fruits, vegetables, nuts, seeds, tofu and whole grains (ideally 100% whole grains) are good choices? When I began my journey into healthful foods, I was not very aware of another food, namely seaweeds. They are the large leafy plants seen in the ocean. The first time I looked for them in the grocery store, in the "seafood" section, which was mostly fish, I found a small section of dried seaweeds. I didn't know what to do with these flat, dried sheets. I have learned to make a few things with them, such as sushi rolls, which are wrapped in them. I usually put a small amount of brown rice, cucumber, avocado and a little avocado-oil mayonnaise onto the flat, dry seaweed sheet, roll everything together, seal it closed with some water along the edge and then enjoy. The seaweeds are also good in soups, stews, and vegetable stir-fry. They sell snack-packs for lunchboxes, too. They are quite nutritious. The seaweeds are a rich source of bioactive compounds not found in the terrestrial plants. [9,10,11,12,13]

So, what is currently known about seaweed and its' contribution to human health? Studies that compared Japanese and Western diets found seaweed linked to lower incidence of chronic diseases such as cancer, coronary heart disease (CHD) and high cholesterol. [9] As previous research has shown that the traditional Asian diet, rich in fish and soy, and low in animal fat and protein, contributes to the reduced occurrence of several chronic diseases, new research has focused on the contribution of seaweed to health. [9] The longest life expectancies in the world are enjoyed by the Japanese, especially the Okinawans.[17] They have a traditional diet composed of fish, soy and seaweed. The consumption of seaweed may be as high as 5.3 g/day in Japan. [9] They enjoy a low incidence of all cancers and from cardiovascular disease (CVD). A more recent review on the health benefits of seaweed consumption notes that seaweed is a nutrient-rich food containing vitamins A, B, C, D, E and K along with essential minerals (calcium, copper, fluoride, iodine, iron, magnesium, manganese, phosphorous, potassium, selenium and zinc), essential amino acids, protein and polyphenols. The polyphenols exhibit anti-inflammatory and anti-oxidant properties. Seaweeds are also rich in healthy polyunsaturated fats.[10,11,12,13] Seaweeds are classified by color, brown, green or red algae and each group has diverse biologically active compounds. For example, the brown seaweeds possess the bioactive compound, fucoidan, which has antibacterial, anti-inflammatory and antiviral effects. They also contain the polyunsaturated fatty acids (PUFAs) linoleic acid (LA), arachidonic acid (AA), docosahexaenoic acid (DHA) and eicosapentaenoic acid (EPA), the essential fatty acids that are found in fish. The seaweeds are in fact, the source of these essential fatty acids; they synthesize these essential omega-3 and omega-6 PUFAs. [13] Also found in brown seaweed are phlorotannins, which protect the seaweeds from stress and UV radiation. The biological activity of the brown seaweeds that are exerted by these phlorotannins include anticancer, antioxidant and anti-inflammatory activities. The red seaweeds produce compounds known as terpenes, and the activities of these compounds include anti-bacterial, anti-cancer and anti-fungal. [11] The green seaweeds contain different PUFAs than the red and brown seaweed, exhibiting the best anti-inflammatory activity, along with monounsaturated fatty acids (MUFAs), which exhibit antioxidant activity. [11,12,13]

So, then, seaweeds are considered a "nutraceutical food," which means they have positive effects on our health. How can one use this knowledge to improve the nutritional status of children? One possibility is to use it as a seasoning. Triple Blend Flakes [14] is a blend of three flaked dried seaweeds, dulse (a red seaweed) laver and sea lettuce (two green seaweeds). It can be sprinkled on all kinds of food, such as popcorn, salads, stir-fry and in soups and gives it a lovely flavor. Also, there is Japanese multi-purpose seasoning, which includes nori. [15] The dried leaves are also sold online in various shapes and sizes. I often buy sheets of nori as snack packs [16] or large sheets at the grocery store, which I use as wraps, instead of sandwich bread.

If you feel my book is helpful to you, it would be much appreciated if you would consider leaving a positive review so that others can more easily find it.

CHAPTER 8: NO ALCOHOL

I am sure by now everyone has heard they should not drink alcohol during pregnancy and yet, worldwide, roughly 10% of pregnant women still do drink, with varying rates, depending on the country. [1] In 1981, the US Surgeon General advised women who were or were considering pregnancy to limit the amount of alcohol consumed. In 2005, the Surgeon General recommended abstinence for these same women, to eliminate the risks of alcohol to a developing fetus. In other words, there is no known safe amount of alcohol consumption for a pregnant woman, even if she does not know yet that she is pregnant. A woman may not yet know she is pregnant and can unintentionally expose the fetus to the adverse effects of alcohol in utero. In addition, alcohol consumption has other adverse effects, such as unstable homes, unstable relationships, violence, and car crashes.[2]

If you have small children in your life, you may not be thinking of alcohol with respect to them. However, alcohol is a common theme in the lives of some adolescents, and indirectly through the adults around them, some children. They need guidance on this topic, since it is everywhere, they may have parents that use (and/or abuse) alcohol, or they may have peer pressure to try it and to use it, even to abuse it. Why would I discuss it here? After all, it is not a food or nutrient; it is in fact, for the most part, a toxin that interferes with proper metabolism. It can impair health. And, for these reasons, I think it is appropriate here. In my introductory nutrition textbook, alcohol is described as having an influence on the brain, the gastrointestinal tract and the liver. The damage done by alcohol includes dehydration and malnutrition. People who drink alcohol urinate more. This can result in dehydration and can be relieved by drinking more water. However, the loss of important minerals, vital to the body's fluid balance, must also be restored. When consumed in moderate doses, alcohol is easily metabolized and thus can contribute to weight gain and increased body fat. The more alcohol that people drink, which, at 7 calories per gram, is calorie-dense, the less likely they are to consume nutrient dense food, and to get the nutrients they need. [3]

The 2020-2025 DGA advises that alcohol should be consumed, if at all, in moderation.[4] Since alcohol supplies calories with few nutrients, one has to know how many drinks are considered 'in moderation' and also, how much is 'a drink'. For adult men, it is recommended that no more than two drinks or less per day are consumed and for adult women, it is no more than one drink or less per day. One alcoholic drink equivalent is (for adults) 12 fluid ounces of regular beer (5% alcohol), 5 fluid ounces of wine (12% alcohol) or 1.5 fluid ounces of 80 proof distilled spirits (40% alcohol). [4] For women who are or may become pregnant, as noted above, there is no safe amount of alcohol consumption. These guidelines are for adults, so, what about adolescents and children?

The American Academy of Pediatrics came out with a policy statement in 2019 [5] in which the potentially adverse effects of underage drinking on the developing brain are discussed. The important thing to note about brain development is that it continues into early adulthood and that exposure to alcohol may impair the maturation of the adolescent brain. For this reason, the National Institute on Alcohol Abuse and Alcoholism recommends that there should be no alcohol use at all before the age of 21 years. In those adolescents using alcohol, deficits have been observed in attention, memory, executive function and information processing, when compared to teenagers that do not. Underage drinking is associated with an increased risk of anxiety, depression, sleep disturbance, suicidal behavior, along with other high-risk behaviors, such as criminal behavior. Also, importantly, the early onset of drinking in adolescence can increase the risk of alcohol use disorder (AUD) in adulthood. While there are several factors that contribute to underage drinking, parental and peer modeling of alcohol use is a significant contributing factor, along with parents who appear tolerant of underage drinking. If an adolescent is aware of their parent's disapproval of underage alcohol consumption, this fact can be a protective factor. So, this response in the parent can contribute to an adolescent's healthy attitude towards alcohol. The good news is that the establishment of the minimum purchase age of 21 years in the United States has resulted in a significant reduction of automobile crash rates for 16 to 17, year-old youths and reduction in the long-term effects of alcohol consumption. [4, 5, 6, 7, 8]

If a woman is not likely to be or become pregnant, and an adolescent has matured to adulthood, alcohol consumption has been shown to be protective or at least not detrimental to the cardiovascular (CV) system in moderate and low amounts of consumption and detrimental to the CV system and to increase the risk of many diseases when consumed in high amounts. [9]

CHAPTER 9: GOOD SLEEP

Up until now, most of what I have written here has been about food and nutrients. So, you might wonder why there are some thoughts on sleep. Well, as it turns out, there is a connection between sleep, nutrition and health. [1] Sleep quality and duration are related to common nutrition-related diseases, such as childhood obesity diabetes, cancer, sleep apnea, and all-cause mortality [2] as well as poor mental health, attention, and behavior problems. It can also affect wound healing. So, what can be done to improve sleep hygiene? Childhood weight status, sleep duration and quality are improved when children do not use electronic entertainment and communication devices (EECD), such as TVs, computers, video games, cell phones and tablets one hour before sleep time. [3] Poor sleep quality activates hormonal responses that increase appetite and food consumption which can lead to obesity. The Center for Disease Control [4] recommends that children aged 6-12 get 9 to 12 hours of sleep at night, while teenagers aged 13-18 need to get 8 to 10 hours of sleep. Creating good 'sleep hygiene' habits in a child can last into adulthood. These good habits might include removing the electronic devices from the sleeping area, avoiding large meals and sugar before bedtime and giving adequate activity during the day to help a child/adolescent fall asleep. Artificial light, especially the blue-enriched, short-wavelength light from computers, tablets and smartphones, is similar to morning sunlight, and can block the 'sleep hormone' melatonin, from being released. This melatonin blockage results in more alertness, and can result in sleep disturbance. [5,6] Two, more recent studies looked at brain development and early sleep patterns. [7,8] Sleep has been shown to affect brain activity, depending on the developmental stage. Before the age of 3, sleep mostly supports learning and reorganization of the neural networks as learning occurs. Sleep, after age 3, is mostly associated with repair and brain 'housekeeping'. These changes may reflect early brain development. Importantly, sleep plays an important role in cognition and cognitive processing. An observational study of 6 to 12-year old children compared participants that were described as having either sufficient sleep or insufficient sleep, with the cutoff being 9 hours of sleep per day. [8] These children were studied for 2 years, looking at mental health, cognition, behavioral problems, and measurement of brain structure and function. The differences between these groups was significant, both in behavioral measures and structure/function measures. The differences in brain structure and function from lack of sleep were instrumental in the resulting differences in depression, stored accumulated knowledge and thought problems. Good sleep, of sufficient duration and well-timed, allows for more successful family relationships, too.

CHAPTER 10: A PREPARED ENVIRONMENT

When my child was young, they were in a Montessori pre-school. One of the foundational tenets of the Montessori method is to create a 'prepared environment', where the child has the freedom to do any of the projects on the shelves, their choice, but the shelves only have projects that are acceptable in the Montessori classroom. [1] In this way, the child can feel independence within the confines of acceptable projects.
This approach can also work in the home, particularly in the kitchen/pantry. Young children are not yet able to drive; the only food available to them is provided to them by the adults in their life. While they may be made aware of ultra-processed foods through marketing, it is up to the adults to guide them, with the foods that are available to them at home and school. When purchasing foods, the nutrition labels can help a parent keep much of added sugar and ultra-processed food, out of their reach. A parent can reduce the quantity of processed meats in the home, highly processed carbohydrates lacking in adequate fiber (ideally, at least, 3 grams per serving), and sugary candy. If they find only healthy foods in the pantry, that is what they will eat. A parent can also limit (or eliminate, if possible) the visits to fast food restaurants, where the foods are high in calories, salt, sugar and processed carbohydrates. If you are worried about the environmental and health costs, you can limit the purchase of red meat and other animal products, so damaging to the environment are these products regarding greenhouse gas production, contamination of water with animal waste, and the welfare of the animals, to name a few concerns. At the same time, unprocessed plant foods including whole grains, vegetables, fruits, beans, and healthy fats such as

avocados, seeds and nuts, can help a child choose the right foods for themselves. Habits start in childhood.

NOTES:

INTRODUCTION NOTES:

1) La Leche League (www.llli.org)

2) White, B. A., Horwath, C. C., & Conner, T. S. (2013). Many apples a day keep the blues away--daily experiences of negative and positive affect and food consumption in young adults. *British journal of health psychology, 18*(4), 782–798. https://doi.org/10.1111/bjhp.12021

3) Blanchflower, D.G., Oswald, A.J. & Stewart-Brown, S. Is Psychological Well-Being   Linked to the Consumption of Fruit and Vegetables?. *Soc Indic   Res* 114, 785–801 (2013). https://doi.org/10.1007/s11205-012-0173-y

4) Mujcic, R., & J Oswald, A. (2016). Evolution of Well-Being and Happiness After Increases in Consumption of Fruit and Vegetables. *American journal of public health*, *106*(8), 1504–1510. https://doi.org/10.2105/AJPH.2016.303260

5) Wahl, D. R., Villinger, K., König, L. M., Ziesemer, K., Schupp, H. T., & Renner, B. (2017). Healthy food choices are happy food choices: Evidence from a real life sample using smartphone based assessments. *Scientific reports*, *7*(1), 17069. https://doi.org/10.1038/s41598-017-17262-9

6)Blumfield, M., Mayr, H., De Vlieger, N., Abbott, K., Starck, C., Fayet-Moore, F., & Marshall, S. (2022). Should We 'Eat a Rainbow'? An Umbrella Review of the Health Effects of Colorful Bioactive Pigments in Fruits and Vegetables. *Molecules (Basel, Switzerland)*, *27*(13), 4061. https://doi.org/10.3390/molecules27134061

7) Minich D. M. (2019). A Review of the Science of Colorful, Plant- Based Food and Practical Strategies for "Eating the Rainbow". *Journal of nutrition and metabolism*, *2019*, 2125070. https://doi.org/10.1155/2019/2125070

BACKGROUND AND METHODS NOTES
1) Furthner, D., Weghuber, D., Dalus, C., Lukas, A.,
    Stundner-Ladenhauf, H. N., Mangge, H., & Pixner, T.
    (2022). Nonalcoholic Fatty Liver Disease in Children with
    Obesity: Narrative Review and Research
    Gaps. *Hormone research in paediatrics*, *95*(2), 167–176.
    https://doi.org/10.1159/000518595

2) Pubmed: https://pubmed.ncbi.nlm.nih.gov/

CHAPTER 1: NUTRITION FACTS LABEL NOTES

1) Food Insight (2020) The Nutrition Facts Label: Its History, Purpose and Updates
   https://foodinsight.org/the-nutrition-facts-label its-history-purpose-and-updates

2) Institute of Medicine (US) Committee on Examination of Front-of-Package Nutrition Rating Systems and Symbols; Wartella EA, Lichtenstein AH, Boon CS, editors. Front-of-Package Nutrition Rating Systems and Symbols: Phase I Report. Washington (DC): National Academies Press (US); 2010. 2, History of Nutrition Labeling. Available from: https://www.ncbi.nlm.nih.gov/books/NBK209859/

3) The New Nutrition Facts Label
   https://www.fda.gov/food/nutrition-education-resources-materials/new-nutrition-facts-label

CHAPTER 2: ESSENTIAL FATTY ACIDS NOTES

1) Crawford, M. A., Bloom, M., Broadhurst, C. L., Schmidt, W. F., Cunnane, S. C., Galli, C., Gehbremeskel, K., Linseisen, F., Lloyd-Smith, J., & Parkington, J. (1999). Evidence for the unique function of docosahexaenoic acid during the evolution of the modern hominid brain. *Lipids, 34 Suppl*, S39–S47. https://doi.org/10.1007/BF02562227

2) _Stetka, Bret on March 1, 2016, Scientific American By Land or by Sea: How Did Early Humans Access Key Brain- Building Nutrients? Experts debate the origins of fatty acids in our ancestors' diets

3) Dhaka, V., Gulia, N., Ahlawat, K. S., & Khatkar, B. S. (2011). Trans fats-sources, health risks and alternative approach - A review. *Journal of food science and technology, 48*(5), 534–541. https://doi.org/10.1007/s13197-010-0225-8

4) Simopoulos A. P. (2006). Evolutionary aspects of diet, the omega-6/omega-3 ratio and genetic variation: nutritional implications for chronic diseases. *Biomedicine & pharmacotherapy = Biomedecine & pharmacotherapie, 60*(9), 502–507. https://doi.org/10.1016/j.biopha.2006.07.080

5) Simopoulos A. P. (2016). An Increase in the Omega-6/Omega-3 Fatty Acid Ratio Increases the Risk for Obesity. *Nutrients*, *8*(3), 128. https://doi.org/10.3390/nu8030128

6) Patterson, E., Wall, R., Fitzgerald, G. F., Ross, R. P., & Stanton, C. (2012). Health implications of high dietary omega-6 polyunsaturated Fatty acids. *Journal of nutrition and metabolism*, *2012*, 539426. https://doi.org/10.1155/2012/539426

7) Ehr, I. J., Persia, M. E., & Bobeck, E. A. (2017). Comparative omega-3 fatty acid enrichment of egg yolks from first-cycle laying hens fed flaxseed oil or ground flaxseed. *Poultry science*, *96*(6), 1791–1799. https://doi.org/10.3382/ps/pew462

8) A P Simopoulos The importance of the ratio of omega-6/omega-3 essential fatty acids Biomed Pharmacotherapy. 2002 Oct;56(8):365-79. PMID: **12442909.** DOI: 10.1016/s0753-3322(02)00253-6

9) Shahidi, F., & Ambigaipalan, P. (2018). Omega-3 Polyunsaturated Fatty Acids and Their Health Benefits. *Annual review of food science and technology*, *9*, 345–381. https://doi.org/10.1146/annurev-food-111317-095850

10) Borderías, A. J., & Sánchez-Alonso, I. (2011). First processing steps and the quality of wild and farmed fish. *Journal of food science, 76*(1), R1–R5. https://doi.org/10.1111/j.1750-3841.2010.01900.x

11) 2022 Cleveland Clinic: Omega-3 Fatty Acids https://my.clevelandclinic.org/health/articles/17290-omega-3-fatty-acids

12) Coletta, J. M., Bell, S. J., & Roman, A. S. (2010). Omega-3 Fatty acids and pregnancy. *Reviews in obstetrics & gynecology, 3*(4), 163–171.

13) DiNicolantonio, J. J., & O'Keefe, J. (2021). The Importance of Maintaining a Low Omega-6/Omega-3 Ratio for Reducing the Risk of Autoimmune Diseases, Asthma, and Allergies. *Missouri medicine, 118*(5), 453–459.

14) Peñalver, R., Lorenzo, J. M., Ros, G., Amarowicz, R., Pateiro, M., & Nieto, G. (2020). Seaweeds as a Functional Ingredient for a Healthy Diet. *Marine drugs, 18*(6), 301. https://doi.org/10.3390/md18060301

15) Harris, W. S., Mozaffarian, D., Rimm, E., Kris-Etherton, P., Rudel, L. L., Appel, L. J., Engler, M. M., Engler, M. B., & Sacks, F. (2009). Omega-6 fatty acids and risk for cardiovascular disease: a science advisory from the American Heart Association Nutrition Subcommittee of the Council on Nutrition, Physical Activity, and Metabolism; Council on Cardiovascular Nursing; and Council on Epidemiology and Prevention. *Circulation, 119*(6), 902–907. https://doi.org/10.1161/CIRCULATIONAHA.108.19162

16) Khaw, K. T., Sharp, S. J., Finikarides, L., Afzal, I., Lentjes, M., Luben, R., & Forouhi, N. G. (2018). Randomised trial of coconut oil, olive oil or butter on blood lipids and other cardiovascular risk factors in healthy men and women. *BMJ open, 8*(3), e020167. https://doi.org/10.1136/bmjopen-2017-020167

17) Rabail, R., Shabbir, M. A., Sahar, A., Miecznikowski, A., Kieliszek, M., & Aadil, R. M. (2021). An Intricate Review on Nutritional and Analytical Profiling of Coconut, Flaxseed, Olive, and Sunflower Oil Blends. *Molecules (Basel, Switzerland), 26*(23), 7187. https://doi.org/10.3390/molecules26237187

19) Carlson, S. E., Colombo, J., Gajewski, B. J., Gustafson, K. M.,
Mundy, D., Yeast, J., Georgieff, M. K., Markley, L. A.,
Kerling, E.   H., & Shaddy, D. J. (2013). DHA
supplementation and pregnancy outcomes. *The American
journal of clinical nutrition*, *97*(4), 808–   815.
https://doi.org/10.3945/ajcn.112.050021

20) Carlson, S. et al. (2021)
Higher dose docosahexaenoic acid supplementation during
pregnancy and early preterm birth: A randomized, double-
blind, adaptive-design superiority trial
https://doi.org/10.1016/j.eclinm.2021.100905

21) Vafai, Y., et al (2022) The association between first trimester
omega-3 fatty acid supplementation and fetal   growth
trajectories. American Journal of Obstetrics and Gynecology
Published August 8, 2022 DOI:
https://doi.org/10.1016/j.ajog.2022.08.007

22) Danielle N Christifano, Lynn Chollet-Hinton, Nicole B Mathis,
Byron J Gajewski, Susan E Carlson, John Colombo, Kathleen
M Gustafson, (2022) DHA Supplementation During Pregnancy
Enhances Maternal Vagally Mediated Cardiac Autonomic
Control in Humans, *The Journal of Nutrition*, 2022;
nxac178, https://doi.org/10.1093/jn/nxac178

23) Carughi, A., Feeney, M.J., Kris-Etherton, P. *et al.* Pairing nuts and dried fruit for cardiometabolic health. *Nutr J* 15, 23 (2015). https://doi.org/10.1186/s12937-016-0142-4

24) Coconut oil: https://www.hsph.harvard.edu/nutritionsource/food-features/coconut-oil/

25) Jasmine F Millman and others, Extra-virgin olive oil and the gut-brain axis: influence on gut microbiota, mucosal immunity, and cardiometabolic and cognitive health, *Nutrition Reviews*, Volume 79, Issue 12, December 2021, Pages 1362–1374, https://doi.org/10.1093/nutrit/nuaa148

26) Chang, C. Y., Ke, D. S., & Chen, J. Y. (2009). Essential fatty acids and human brain. *Acta neurologica Taiwanica*, *18*(4), 231–241

27) Chianese, R., Coccurello, R., Viggiano, A., Scafuro, M., Fiore, M., Coppola, G., Operto, F. F., Fasano, S., Laye, S., Pierantoni, R., & Meccariello, R. (2018). Impact of Dietary Fats on Brain Functions. *Current neuropharmacology*, *16*(7), 1059–1085. https://doi.org/10.2174/1570159X15666171017102547

28) Dietary Guidelines for Americans (2020-2025) https://www.dietaryguidelines.gov/resources/2020-2025-dietary-guidelines-online-materials

29) Poli A, Agostoni C, Visioli F. Dietary Fatty Acids and Inflammation: Focus on the n-6 Series. *International Journal of Molecular Sciences*. 2023; 24(5):4567. https://doi.org/10.3390/ijms24054567

30) Sneh Punia, Kawaljit Singh Sandhu, Anil Kumar Siroha, Sanju Bala Dhull, Omega 3-metabolism, absorption, bioavailability and health benefits–A review, PharmaNutrition, Volume 10, 2019, 100162, ISSN 2213-4344, https://doi.org/10.1016/j.phanu.2019.100162

CHAPTER 3: BREASTFEEDING IS BEST NOTES:

1) _Dieterich, C.M., BS, MS, RD, _Felice, J.P. BS, O'Sullivan, E.,BA, BS, and _Rasmussen, K.M., AB, ScM, ScD, R. Breastfeeding and Health Outcomes for the Mother-Infant Dyad Pediatr Clin North Am. 2013 Feb; 60(1): 31–48. doi: 10.1016/j.pcl.2012.09.010

2) Colin Binns, MBBS, PhD, MiKyung Lee, MA, PhD, and Wah Yun Low, PhD The Long-Term Public Health Benefits of Breastfeeding Volume 28, Issue 1_First published online January 20, 2016 https://doi.org/10.1177/1010539515624964

3) Schwarz, 2015 Schwarz, E.B., MD, MS, Nothnagle, M., MD, MSC, The Maternal Health Benefits of Breastfeeding *Am. Fam. Physician.* 2015;91(9):602-604

4) North, K., MD, MPH Gao, M., MD, Allen, G., Lee, Anne., MD, MPH. Breastfeeding in a Global Context: Epidemiology, Impact, and Future Directions. REVIEW| VOLUME 44, ISSUE 2, P228-244, FEBRUARY 01, 2022 DOI: https://doi.org/10.1016/j.clinthera.2021.11.017

5) https://www.ncsl.org/health/breastfeeding-state-laws

6) www.elvie.com

7) www.fetalplus.com

8) www.mon-lait.com

9) La Leche League International www.llli.org

10) Sheila M Innis Impact of maternal diet on human milk composition and neurological development of infants *The American Journal of Clinical Nutrition*, Volume 99, Issue 3, March 2014, Pages 734S-741S, https://doi.org/10.3945/ajcn.113.072595 Published: 05 February 2014

11) Di Maso, 2022 Di Maso, M., et al. (2022). Adherence to Mediterranean Diet of Breastfeeding Mothers and Fatty Acids Composition of Their Human Milk: Results From the Italian MEDIDIET Study. *Frontiers in nutrition*, *9*, 891376. https://doi.org/10.3389/fnut.2022.891376

12) Susana Figueroa-Lozano, Paul de Vos (2018) Relationship Between Oligosaccharides and Glycoconjugates Content in Human Milk and the Development of the Gut Barrier Comprehensive Reviews in Food Science and Food Safety 25 October 2018 https://doi.org/10.1111/1541-4337.12400

13) https://www.myplate.gov/life-stages/pregnancy-and-breastfeeding

14) Ford, E. L., Underwood, M. A., & German, J. B. (2020). Helping Mom Help Baby: Nutrition-Based Support for the Mother-Infant Dyad During Lactation. *Frontiers in nutrition*, 7, 54. https://doi.org/10.3389/fnut.2020.00054

15) Martin, C. R., Ling, P. R., & Blackburn, G. L. (2016). Review of Infant Feeding: Key Features of Breast Milk and Infant Formula. *Nutrients*, *8*(5), 279. https://doi.org/10.3390/nu8050279

16) Yvan Vandenplas, Badriul Hegar, Zakiudin Munasir, Made Astawan, Mohammad Juffrie, Saptawati Bardosono, Rini Sekartini, Ray Wagiu Basrowi, Erika Wasito,
The role of soy plant-based formula supplemented with dietary fiber to support children's growth and development: An expert opinion,
Nutrition, Volume 90, 2021, 111278, ISSN 0899-9007,
https://doi.org/10.1016/j.nut.2021.111278

17) https://www.urmc.rochester.edu/childrens-hospital/breastfeeding-lactation-medicine.aspx
Rochester Review, Fall 2022, University of Rochester, Rochester, NY

CHAPTER 4: GUT HEALTH, FIBER AND FERMENTED FOODS NOTES:

1) Ramirez, J. et al. (2020)
Antibiotics as Major Disruptors of Gut Microbiota. Front Cell Infect Microbiol. 2020; 10: 572912.
Published online 2020 Nov24. doi: 10.3389/fcimb.2020.572912

2) Ma, J., Qiao, Y., Zhao, P., Li, W., Katzmarzyk, P. T., Chaput, J. P., Fogelholm, M., Kuriyan, R., Lambert, E. V., Maher, C., Maia, J., Matsudo, V., Olds, T., Onywera, V., Sarmiento, O. L., 3Standage, M., Tremblay, M. S., Tudor-Locke, C., Hu, G., & ISCOLE Research Group (2020). Breastfeeding and childhood obesity: A 12-country study. *Maternal & child nutrition*, *16*(3), e12984. https://doi.org/10.1111/mcn.12984

3) Sobko, T., Liang, S., Cheng, W. H. G., & Tun, H. M. (2020). Impact of outdoor nature-related activities on gut microbiota, fecal serotonin, and perceived stress in preschool children: the Play&Grow randomized controlled trial. *Scientific reports*, *10*(1), 21993. https://doi.org/10.1038/s41598-020-78642-2

4) Amir, A., Erez-Granat, O., Braun, T., Sosnovski, K., Hadar, R., BenShoshan, M., Heiman, S., Abbas-Egbariya, H., Glick Saar, E., Efroni, G., & Haberman, Y. (2022). Gut microbiome development in early childhood is affected by day care attendance. *NPJ biofilms and microbiomes*, *8*(1), 2. https://doi.org/10.1038/s41522-021-00265-w

5) Sanchez, G. V., Fleming-Dutra, K. E., Roberts, R. M., &
Hicks, L. A. (2016). Core Elements of Outpatient Antibiotic
Stewardship. *MMWR. Recommendations and reports:
Morbidity and mortality weekly report. Recommendations and
reports*, *65*(6), 1–12. https://doi.org/10.15585/mmwr.rr6506a1

6) King, L. M., Fleming-Dutra, K. E., & Hicks, L. A. (2018).
Advances in optimizing the prescription of antibiotics in
outpatient settings. *BMJ (Clinical research ed.)*, *363*, k3047.
https://doi.org/10.1136/bmj.k3047

7) D'Yans, M. "Garden in Your Belly" Publisher: Millbrook
Press, 2020

8) Brasnan, Katie "Gut Garden" Publisher: Cicada Books, 2020

9) Davies, Sean and Tori "The Incredible Microbiome" Publisher:
Davies, S 2018

10) Dr. Seuss. "Green Eggs and Ham", Publisher: Random House,
1960

11) Child, L. "I Will Never Not Ever Eat a Tomato" Publisher:
Candlewick Books 2003

12) Berenstain, J. and S. "Too Much Junk Food", Publisher: Random House Books, New York, NY 1985

13) Ceylani, T., Jakubowska-Doğru, E., Gurbanov, R., Teker, H. T., & Gozen, A. G. (2018). The effects of repeated antibiotic administration to juvenile BALB/c mice on the microbiota status and animal behavior at the adult age. *Heliyon*, *4*(6), e00644. https://doi.org/10.1016/j.heliyon.2018.e00644

14) McNamara, M., et al. (2021)
Early-life effects of juvenile Western diet and exercise on adult gut microbiome composition in mice. Journal of Experimental Biology (2021) 224 (4): jeb239699
https://doi.org/10.1242/jeb.239699

15) Bruno Senghor, Cheikh Sokhna, Raymond Ruimy, Jean-Christophe Lagier,
Gut microbiota diversity according to dietary habits and geographical provenance, Human Microbiome Journal, Volumes 7–8, 2018, Pages   1-9
https://doi.org/10.1016/j.humic.2018.01.001

16) Kranz, S., et al. (2012).
What do we know about dietary fiber intake in children and health? The effects of fiber intake on constipation, obesity, and diabetes in children. *Advances in nutrition (Bethesda, Md.)*, *3*(1), 47–53. https://doi.org/10.3945/an.111.001362

17) Hojsak, I., Benninga, M. A., Hauser, B., Kansu, A., Kelly, V. B., Stephen, A. M., Morais Lopez, A., Slavin, J., & Tuohy, K. (2022). Benefits of dietary fibre for children in health and disease. *Archives of disease in childhood, 107*(11), 973–979. https://doi.org/10.1136/archdischild-2021-323571

18) Singh, R.K., Chang, HW., Yan, D. *et al.* Influence of diet on the gut microbiome and implications for human health. *J Transl Med* 15, 73 (2017). https://doi.org/10.1186/s12967-017-1175-y

19) Atkinson, F. S., Foster-Powell, K., & Brand-Miller, J. C. (2008). International tables of glycemic index (GI) and glycemic load (GL) values: 2008. *Diabetes care, 31*(12), 2281–2283. https://doi.org/10.2337/dc08-1239

20) Bahado-Singh, P. S., Riley, C. K., Wheatley, A. O., & Lowe, H. I. (2011). Relationship between Processing Method and the Glycemic Indices of Ten Sweet Potato (Ipomoea batatas) Cultivars Commonly Consumed in Jamaica. *Journal of nutrition and metabolism, 2011*, 584832. https://doi.org/10.1155/2011/584832

21) Chan, Y. K., Estaki, M., & Gibson, D. L. (2013). Clinical consequences of diet-induced dysbiosis. *Annals of nutrition & metabolism, 63 Suppl 2*, 28–40. https://doi.org/10.1159/000354902

22) Dueñas, 2015 Cueva, Ana Jiménez-Girón, Fernando Sánchez-Patán, Celestino Santos-Buelga, M. Victoria Moreno-Arribas, and **Begoña Bartolomé**
A Survey of Modulation of Gut Microbiota by Dietary Polyphenols **BioMed Research International**
Volume 2015 | ArticleID 850902 |
https://doi.org/10.1155/2015/850902

23) Mark L. Heiman, Frank L. Greenway,
A healthy gastrointestinal microbiome is dependent on dietary diversity,
Molecular Metabolism, Volume 5, Issue 5, 2016, Pages 317-320,
ISSN 2212-8778,
https://doi.org/10.1016/j.molmet.2016.02.005.

24) Edwards, C. A., Havlik, J., Cong, W., Mullen, W., Preston, T., Morrison, D. J., & Combet, E. (2017).   Polyphenols and health: Interactions   between fibre, plant polyphenols and the gut microbiota. *Nutrition   bulletin*, *42*(4), 356–360.
https://doi.org/10.1111/nbu.12296

25) www.medlineplus.gov

26) Wastyk, H.C. et al. 2021. Gut-microbiota-targeted diets modulate human immune status Cell vol. 184, pgs. 4137-4153
https://doi.org/10.1016/j.cell.2021.06.019

1) A) Shiza Arshad, Tahniat Rehman, Summaya Saif, Muhammad Shahid Riaz Rajoka, Muhammad Modassar Ali Nawaz Ranjha, Abdo Hassoun, Janna Cropotova, Monica Trif, Aqsa Younas, Rana Muhammad Aadil,
Replacement of refined sugar by natural sweeteners: focus on potential health benefits,
Heliyon, Volume 8, Issue 9, 2022, e10711, ISSN 2405-8440,
https://doi.org/10.1016/j.heliyon.2022.e10711.

B) Sabra, A., Netticadan, T., & Wijekoon, C. (2021). Grape bioactive molecules, and the potential health benefits in reducing the risk of heart diseases. *Food chemistry: X, 12,* 100149. https://doi.org/10.1016/j.fochx.2021.100149

2) Tsan, L., et al. (2022) Early-life low-calorie sweetener consumption disrupts glucose regulation, sugar-motivated behavior, and memory function in rats JCI Insight, 10.1172/jci.insight.157714

3) Suez, J.,et. al.(2022). Personalized microbiome-driven effects of non-nutritive sweeteners on human glucose tolerance. *Cell, 185*(18), 3307–3328.e19.
https://doi.org/10.1016/j.cell.2022.07.016

4) Stamataki, N. S., Crooks, B., Ahmed, A., & McLaughlin, J. T. (2020). Effects of the Daily Consumption of Stevia on Glucose Homeostasis, Body Weight, and Energy Intake: A Randomised Open-Label 12-Week Trial in Healthy Adults. *Nutrients*, *12*(10), 3049. https://doi.org/10.3390/nu12103049

5) Peteliuk, V., Rybchuk, L., Bayliak, M., Storey, K. B., & Lushchak, O. (2021). Natural sweetener *Stevia rebaudiana*: Functionalities, health benefits and potential risks. *EXCLI journal*, *20*, 1412–1430. https://doi.org/10.17179/excli2021-4211

6) DGA, 2020-2025 Dietary Guidelines for Americans: https://www.dietaryguidelines.gov/sites/default/files/2020-12/Dietary_Guidelines_for_Americans_2020-2025.pdf

7) Krebs-Smith, S. M., Guenther, P. M., Subar, A. F., Kirkpatrick, S. I., & Dodd, K. W. (2010). Americans do not meet federal dietary recommendations. *The Journal of nutrition*, *140*(10), 1832–1838. https://doi.org/10.3945/jn.110.124826

8) Grimm, K. A., Kim, S. A., Yaroch, A. L., & Scanlon, K. S. (2014). Fruit and vegetable intake during infancy and early childhood. *Pediatrics*, *134 Suppl 1*(Suppl 1), S63–S69. https://doi.org/10.1542/peds.2014-0646K

9) Calvano, A., Izuora, K., , Oh, E. C., , Ebersole, J. L., , Lyons, T. J., & Basu, A., (2019). Dietary berries, insulin resistance and type 2 diabetes: an overview of human feeding trials. *Food & function*, *10*(10), 6227–6243. https://doi.org/10.1039/c9fo01426h

10) Basaranoglu, M., Basaranoglu, G., & Bugianesi, E. (2015). Carbohydrate intake and nonalcoholic fatty liver disease: fructose as a weapon of mass destruction. Hepatobiliary surgery and nutrition, 4(2), 109–116. https://doi.org/10.3978/j.issn.2304-3881.2014.11.05

11) Jang, C., Wada, S., Yang, S. *et al.* The small intestine shields the liver from fructose-induced steatosis. *Nat Metab* 2, 586–593 (2020). https://doi.org/10.1038/s42255-020-0222-9

12) Jensen, T., Abdelmalek, M., Sullivan, S., Nadeau, K., Green, M., Roncal, C., Nakagawa, T., Kuwabara, M., Sato, Y., Kang, D., Tolan, D., Sanchez-Lozada, L., Rosen, H., Lanaspa, M., Diehl, A., Johnson, R.
Fructose and sugar: A major mediator of non-alcoholic fatty liver   disease
REVIEW| VOLUME 68, ISSUE 5, P1063-1075, MAY 2018.
JOURNAL OF HEPATOLOGY Published: February 03, 2018
DOI: https://doi.org/10.1016/j.jhep.2018.01.019

CHAPTER 6: A HEALTHY LIFESTYLE

1) O'Neil, C. E., Nicklas, T. A., & Fulgoni, V. L., 3rd (2018). Food Sources of Energy and Nutrients of Public Health Concern and Nutrients to Limit with a Focus on Milk and other Dairy Foods in Children 2 to 18 Years of Age: National Health and Nutrition Examination Survey, 2011⁻2014. *Nutrients, 10*(8), 1050. https://doi.org/10.3390/nu10081050

2) AMA (American Medical Association), 2018 Culturally Responsive Dietary and Nutritional Guidelines D-440.978: https://policysearch.ama-assn.org/policyfinder/detail/D-440.978

3) PCRM: https://www.pcrm.org/good-nutrition/nutrition-programs-policies/2020-2025-dietary-guidelines

4) ACS, 2022 https://www.acs.org/pressroom/newsreleases/2022/august/completing-the-micronutrient-picture-for-plant-based-milk-alternatives.html

5) Pires, V., et. al. (2023). Market Basket Survey of the Micronutrients Vitamin A, Vitamin D, Calcium, and Potassium in Eight Types of Commercial Plant-Based Milk Alternatives from United States Markets. *ACS food science & technology, 3*(1), 100–112. https://doi.org/10.1021/acsfoodscitech.2c00317

6) Melnik B. Milk consumption: aggravating factor of acne and promoter of chronic diseases of Western societies, 30 March 2009 Journal of the German Society of Dermatology https://doi.org/10.1111/j.1610-0387.2009.07019.x

7) Larnkjær, A., Arnberg, K., Michaelsen, K. F., Jensen, S. M., & Mølgaard, C. (2014). Effect of milk proteins on linear growth and IGF variables in overweight adolescents. *Growth hormone & IGF research : official journal of the Growth Hormone Research Society and the International IGF Research Society*, *24*(2-3), 54–59. https://doi.org/10.1016/j.ghir.2013.12.004

8) Mullins, A. P., & Arjmandi, B. H. (2021). Health Benefits of Plant-Based Nutrition: Focus on Beans in Cardiometabolic Diseases. *Nutrients*, *13*(2), 519. https://doi.org/10.3390/nu13020519

9) Amparo Sahuquillo, Reyes Barberá, Rosaura Farré Bioaccessibility of calcium, iron and zinc from three legume samples Food / Nahrung Volume 47, Issue 6 p. 438-441 27 November 2003 https://doi.org/10.1002/food.200390097

10) Graham, M., Clark, C., Scherer, A., Ratner, M., & Keen, C. (2023). An Analysis of the Nutritional Adequacy of Mass-Marketed Vegan Recipes. *Cureus*, *15*(4), e37131. https://doi.org/10.7759/cureus.37131

11) Papanikolaou, Y., & Fulgoni, V. L., 3rd (2023). Dairy Food Consumption Is Associated with Reduced Risk of Heart Disease Mortality, but Not All-Cause and Cancer Mortality in US Adults. *Nutrients*, *15*(2), 394. https://doi.org/10.3390/nu15020394

12) Morgan E. Levine, et al.
Low Protein Intake Is Associated with a Major Reduction in IGF-1, Cancer, and Overall Mortality in the 65 and Younger but Not Older Population,
Cell Metabolism, Volume 19, Issue 3, 2014, Pages 407-417, ISSN 1550-4131,
https://doi.org/10.1016/j.cmet.2014.02.006.

13) Milk Intake in Early Life and Later Cancer Risk: A Meta-Analysis
Hyeonmin Gil, Qiao-Yi Chen, Jaewon Khil, Jihyun Park, Gyumi Na,
Donghoon Lee and Nana Keum
Nutrients 2022, *14*(6),
1233; https://doi.org/10.3390/nu14061233

14) Virto M, Santamarina-García G, Amores G, Hernández I. Antibiotics in Dairy Production: Where Is the Problem? *Dairy*. 2022; 3(3):541-564. https://doi.org/10.3390/dairy3030039

15) Al-Shaar, L., Satija, A., Wang, D., Rimm, E, Smith-Warner, S.A., Stampfer, M., Hu, Frank., Willett, W.C. (2020) Red meat intake and risk of coronary heart disease among US men: prospective cohort study *BMJ* 2020; 371 doi: https://doi.org/10.1136/bmj.m4141

16) Frank Qian,[1,2] Matthew C. Riddle,[3] Judith Wylie-Rosett,[4] and Frank B. Hu[1,5,6]Red and Processed Meats and Health Risks: How Strong Is the Evidence? Diabetes Care. 2020 Feb; 43(2): 265–271. Published online 2020 Jan 13.
doi: 10.2337/dci19-0063

17) Geiker, N. R. W.,et. al.. (2021). Meat and Human Health-Current Knowledge and Research Gaps. *Foods (Basel, Switzerland)*, *10*(7), 1556. https://doi.org/10.3390/foods10071556

18) Omaye, A. T., & Omaye, S. T. (2019). Caveats for the Good and Bad of Dietary Red Meat. *Antioxidants (Basel, Switzerland)*, *8*(11), 544. https://doi.org/10.3390/antiox8110544

19) Prasad., et al. Glycation End Products and Risks for Chronic Diseases: Intervening Through Lifestyle Modification. *American journal of lifestyle medicine*, 2017 *13*(4), 384–404. https://doi.org/10.1177/1559827617708991

20) Rodríguez, J. M., Leiva Balich, L., Concha, M. J., Mizón, C., Bunout Barnett, D., Barrera Acevedo, G., Hirsch Birn, S., Jiménez Jaime, T., Henríquez, S., Uribarri, J., & de la Maza Cave, M. P. (2015). Reduction of serum advanced glycation end-products with a low-calorie Mediterranean diet. *Nutricion hospitalaria*, *31*(6), 2511–2517. https://doi.org/10.3305/nh.2015.31.6.8936

21) Ramírez-Garza, S. L., Laveriano-Santos, E. P., Marhuenda-Muñoz, M., Storniolo, C. E., Tresserra-Rimbau, A., Vallverdú-Queralt, A., & Lamuela-Raventós, R. M. (2018). Health Effects of Resveratrol: Results from Human Intervention Trials. *Nutrients*, *10*(12), 1892. https://doi.org/10.3390/nu10121892

22) Pezzuto, J.M. (2019) Resveratrol: Twenty Years of Growth, Development and   Controversy Biomolecules & Therapeutics 2019; 27(1): 1-14 https://doi.org/10.4062/biomolther.2018.176

23) Serra-Majem, L., Tomaino, L., Dernini, S., Berry, E. M., Lairon, D., Ngo de la Cruz, J., Bach-Faig, A., Donini, L. M., Medina, F. X., Belahsen, R., Piscopo, S., Capone, R., Aranceta-Bartrina, J., La Vecchia, C., & Trichopoulou, A. (2020). Updating the Mediterranean Diet Pyramid towards Sustainability: Focus on Environmental Concerns. *International journal of environmental research and public health*, *17*(23), 8758. https://doi.org/10.3390/ijerph17238758

24) Flori, L., Donnini, S., Calderone, V., Zinnai, A., Taglieri, I., Venturi, F., & Testai, L. (2019). The Nutraceutical Value of Olive Oil and Its Bioactive Constituents on the Cardiovascular System. Focusing on Main Strategies to Slow Down Its Quality Decay during Production and Storage. *Nutrients*, *11*(9), 1962. https://doi.org/10.3390/nu11091962

25) Micha R, Peñalvo JL, Cudhea F, Imamura F, Rehm CD, Mozaffarian D. Association Between Dietary Factors and Mortality From Heart Disease, Stroke, and Type 2 Diabetes in the United States. *JAMA*. 2017;317(9):912–924. https://doi:10.1001/jama.2017.0947

26) Rothpletz-Puglia, P., Fredericks, L., Dreker, M., Patusco, R, Ziegler, J. Position of the Society for Nutrition Education and Behavior: Healthful Food For Children is the Same as Adults Journal of Nutrition Education and Behavior vol. 64 Issue 1 pages 4-11 Jan. 2022. https://doi.org/10.1016/j.jneb.2021.09.007

27) Franks, P. W., Hanson, R. L., Knowler, W. C., Sievers, M. L., Bennett, P. H., & Looker, H. C. (2010). Childhood obesity, other cardiovascular risk factors, and premature death. *The New England journal of medicine*, *362*(6), 485–493. https://doi.org/10.1056/NEJMoa0904130

28) Kaikkonen, 2012 ,Markus Juonala,Jorma S. A. Viikari &Olli
T. Raitakari Does childhood nutrition influence adult
cardiovascular disease risk?—Insights from the Young Finns
Study Pages 120-128 | Received 02 Nov 2011, Accepted 15
Feb 2012, Published online: 12 Apr 2012 Annals of Medicine
https://doi.org/10.3109/07853890.2012.671537

29) Wood, A. C., Blissett, J. M., Brunstrom, J. M., Carnell, S.,
Faith, M. S., Fisher, J. O., Hayman, L. L., Khalsa, A. S.,
Hughes, S. O., Miller, A. L., Momin, S. R., Welsh, J. A., Woo,
J. G., Haycraft, E., & American Heart Association Council on
Lifestyle and Cardiometabolic Health; Council on
Epidemiology and Prevention; Council on Lifelong Congenital
Heart Disease and Heart Health in the Young; Council on
Cardiovascular and Stroke Nursing; and Stroke Council
(2020). Caregiver Influences on Eating Behaviors in Young
Children: A Scientific Statement From the American Heart
Association. *Journal of the American Heart Association*, 9(10),
e014520. https://doi.org/10.1161/JAHA.119.014520

CHAPTER 7: NUTRITIOUS FOODS NOTES

1) Davis, D. R., Epp, M. D., & Riordan, H. D. (2004). Changes in USDA food composition data for 43 garden crops, 1950 to 1999. *Journal of the American College of Nutrition, 23*(6), 669–682. https://doi.org/10.1080/07315724.2004.10719409

2) Davis, D. R. (2009). Declining Fruit and Vegetable Nutrient Composition: What Is the Evidence?. *HortScience horts, 44*(1), 15-19. Retrieved Jul 30, 2023, from https://doi.org/10.21273/HORTSCI.44.1.15

3) Irakli Loladze (2014)
Hidden shift of the ionome of plants exposed to elevated CO_2 depletes minerals at the base of human nutrition
eLife 3:e02245.
https://doi.org/10.7554/eLife.02245

4) Harrington, S.A., et al. A two-gene strategy increases iron and zinc concentrations in wheat flour, improving mineral bioaccessibility, *Plant Physiology*, Volume 191, Issue 1, January 2023, Pages 528–541, https://doi.org/10.1093/plphys/kiac499

5) Montgomery, D.R., Bikle, A. (2016). "The Hidden Half of Nature", the Microbial Roots of Life and Health. W. W. Norton & Company, Inc. New York, NY

6) Thapa, D. B., et al. (2022). Variation in Grain Zinc and Iron Concentrations, Grain Yield and Associated Traits of Biofortified Bread Wheat Genotypes in Nepal. *Frontiers in plant science*, *13*, June 2022. https://doi.org/10.3389/fpls.2022.881965

7) Govindan, V., et al. Crop Science
Volume 62, Issue 5 p. 1912-1925
Breeding increases grain yield, zinc, and iron, supporting enhanced wheat biofortification. First published: 06 May 2022 https://doi.org/10.1002/csc2.20759

8) Montgomery, D. and Bikle, A. Soil Heal, and Nutrient Density: Beyond Organic vs. Conventional Farming. Front. Sustain. Food Syst., 04 November 2021 Sec. Nutrition and Sustainable Diets
Volume 5 - 2021 | https://doi.org/10.3389/fsufs.2021.699147

9) Brown, E. S., Allsopp, P. J., Magee, P. J., Gill, C. I., Nitecki, S., Strain, C. R., & McSorley, E. M. (2014). Seaweed and human health. *Nutrition reviews*, *72*(3), 205–216. https://doi.org/10.1111/nure.12091

10) Swinimer, A. (2021) "The Science and Spirit of Seaweed" Harbour Publishing Company , Madeira Park, BC (Canada)

11) Lomartire, S., Marques, J. C., & Gonçalves, A. M. M. (2021). An Overview to the Health Benefits of Seaweeds Consumption. *Marine drugs*, *19*(6), 341. https://doi.org/10.3390/md19060341

12) Peñalver, R., Lorenzo, J. M., Ros, G., Amarowicz, R., Pateiro, M., & Nieto, G. (2020). Seaweeds as a Functional Ingredient for a Healthy Diet. *Marine drugs*, *18*(6), 301. https://doi.org/10.3390/md18060301

13) Rocha, C. P., Pacheco, D., Cotas, J., Marques, J. C., Pereira, L., & Gonçalves, A. M. M. (2021). Seaweeds as Valuable Sources of Essential Fatty Acids for Human Nutrition. *International journal of environmental research and public health*, *18*(9), 4968. https://doi.org/10.3390/ijerph18094968

14) Maine Coast Sea Vegetables, Inc. Hancock, Maine 04640 (www.seaveg.com)

15) Japanese multi-purpose seasoning, Trader Joe's Monrovia, Ca (www.traderjoe's.com)

16) Costco (www.costco.com)

17) <u>S Miyagi</u>, <u>N Iwama</u>, <u>T Kawabata</u>, <u>K Hasegawa</u> Longevity and diet in Okinawa, Japan: the past, present and future Asia Pac J Public Health. 2003;15 Suppl:S3-9. PMID: 18924533 DOI: <u>10.1177/101053950301500S03</u>

CHAPTER 8: NO ALCOHOL. NOTES

1) Tsang, T.W. & Elliott, E.J. High global prevalence of alcohol use during pregnancy and fetal alcohol syndrome indicates need for urgent action. The Lancet volume 5, Issue 3, E232-E233, March 2017. doi:https://doi.org/10.1016/S2214-109X(17)30008-6

2) DeJong, Wm. _Ph.D., and Blanchette, J. M.P.H.
Case Closed: Research Evidence on the Positive Public Health Impact of the Age 21 Minimum Legal Drinking Age in the United States *Journal of Studies on Alcohol and Drugs, Supplement,* (s17), 108–115 (2014).
https://doi.org/10.15288/jsads.2014.s17.108

3) Rolfes, S.R., Pinna, K., Whitney, E. Nutrition, 10th edition, 2015. Cengage Learning.

4) DGA (2020-2025): Dietary Guidelines for Americans:
https://www.dietaryguidelines.gov/sites/default/files/2020-12/Dietary_Guidelines_for_Americans_2020-2025.pdf

5) Quigley, J. (2019) Alcohol Use by Youth. American Academy of Pediatrics Policy Statement July 1, 2019. *Pediatrics* (2019) 144 (1): e20191356.
https://doi.org/10.1542/peds.2019-1356

6) Voas, R. B., Tippetts, A. S., & Fell, J. (1999). The United States Limits Drinking by Youth Under Age 21: Does this Reduce Fatal Crash Involvements? *Annual Proceedings / Association for the Advancement of Automotive Medicine*, *43*, 265–278

7) Norberg, K. E., Bierut, L. J., & Grucza, R. A. (2009). Long-term effects of minimum drinking age laws on past-year alcohol and drug use disorders. *Alcoholism, clinical and experimental research*, *33*(12), 2180–2190. https://doi.org/10.1111/j.1530-0277.2009.01056.x

8) Rehm, Jurgen. Minimum legal drinking age—still an underrated alcohol control policy. THE LANCET PUBLIC HEALTH COMMENT | VOLUME 8, ISSUE 5, E321-E322, MAY 2023 https://doi.org/10.1016/S2468-2667(23)00054-3

9) Chiva-Blanch, G., & Badimon, L. (2019). Benefits and Risks of Moderate Alcohol Consumption on Cardiovascular Disease: Current Findings and Controversies. *Nutrients*, *12*(1), 108. https://doi.org/10.3390/nu12010108

CHAPTER 9: GOOD SLEEP

1) Du, C., Tucker, R. M., & Yang, C. L. (2023). How Are You Sleeping? Why Nutrition Professionals Should Ask Their Patients About Sleep Habits. *Journal of the American Nutrition Association, 42*(3), 263–273. https://doi.org/10.1080/07315724.2022.2025547

2) Irish, L. A., Kline, C. E., Gunn, H. E., Buysse, D. J., & Hall, M. H. (2015). The role of sleep hygiene in promoting public health: A review of empirical evidence. *Sleep medicine reviews, 22*, 23–36. https://doi.org/10.1016/j.smrv.2014.10.001

3) Dube, N., Khan, K., Loehr, S., Chu, Y., & Veugelers, P. (2017). The use of entertainment and communication technologies before sleep could affect sleep and weight status: a population-based study among children. *The international journal of behavioral nutrition and physical activity, 14*(1), 97. https://doi.org/10.1186/s12966-017-0547-2

4) **CDC:** Learn more about good sleep habits at www.cdc.gov/sleep

5) Qanash, S., Al-Husayni, F., Falata, H., Halawani, O., Jahra, E., Murshed, B., Alhejaili, F., Ghabashi, A., & Alhashmi, H. (2021). Effect of Electronic Device Addiction on Sleep Quality and Academic Performance Among Health Care Students: Cross-sectional Study. *JMIR medical education, 7*(4), e25662. https://doi.org/10.2196/25662

6) Pham, H. T., Chuang, H. L., Kuo, C. P., Yeh, T. P., & Liao, W. C. (2021). Electronic Device Use before Bedtime and Sleep Quality among University Students. *Healthcare (Basel, Switzerland), 9*(9), 1091. https://doi.org/10.3390/healthcare9091091

7) Lokhandwala, S., & Spencer, R. M. C. (2022). Relations between sleep patterns early in life and brain development: A review. *Developmental cognitive neuroscience, 56*, 101130. https://doi.org/10.1016/j.dcn.2022.101130

8) Yang, F. N., Xie, W., & Wang, Z. (2022). Effects of sleep duration on neurocognitive development in early adolescents in the USA: a propensity score matched, longitudinal, observational study. *The Lancet. Child & adolescent health, 6*(10), 705–712. https://doi.org/10.1016/S2352-4642(22)00188-2

CHAPTER 10: A PREPARED ENVIRONMENT NOTES

1) American Montessori Society, 2023
    https://amshq.org/About-Montessori/What-Is-Montessori

INDEX

Ann P. Endal has has worked in numerous laboratory settings (mostly, cancer) in Biology for almost four decades (both research and clinical) before embarking ten years ago on her child caregiver work. This triggered her interest in this topic, child wellness and happiness. She has MS degrees in both Biotechnology, which seeks to use whatever bio-techniques work to improve health and well-being, and Integrative Nutrition, which combines Western understanding of nutrition with traditional nutrition (herbs and plants) to improve nutrition. She has raised her own child to adulthood and lives with her family in the Pacific Northwest.